D1179433

Causation and Disease

A Chronological Journey

Causation and Disease

A Chronological Journey

Alfred S. Evans
Yale University
New Haven, Connecticut

Plenum Medical Book Company
New York and London

Library of Congress Cataloging-in-Publication Data

Evans, Alfred S., 1917-
    Causation and disease : a chronological journey / Alfred S. Evans.
        p.   cm.
    Includes bibliographical references and index.
    ISBN 0-306-44283-3
    1. Diseases--Causes and theories of causation--History.
I. Title.
    [DNLM: 1. Disease--etiology. 2. Epidemiology--history.   WA 11.1
E92c 1993]
RB151.E93   1993
616.07'1--dc20
DNLM/DLC
for Library of Congress   92-48333
                                                                         CIP

ISBN 0-306-44283-3

© 1993 Plenum Publishing Corporation
233 Spring Street, New York, N.Y. 10013

Plenum Medical Book Company is an imprint of Plenum Publishing Corporation

Printed in the United States of America

With love to my children, John, Barbara, and Christopher, and to their families

Foreword

In the front material of this book both a foreword and a preface appear. What the content of a preface should be is well understood. It is the author's retrospective account of intent, of the labors to accomplish that intent, and of the content of the book that resulted. What a foreword should be is less obvious. Most properly, it is perhaps the brief testimony of one who knows the accomplishments of the author and the scope of the field and who may direct readers to the book. On some basis, the writer is assumed to have earned the right to undertake such a task. To undertake the writing of a foreword for so considerable a researcher, teacher, and scholar as Alfred Evans can be seen not only as an honor but also as a daunting one. My first thought, in truth, is that this wine needs no blush and that no foreword is needed.

As John Rodman Paul Professor of Epidemiology at Yale, Alfred Evans has an established reputation in the field of causality. We have learned from his insights about the evolution of causal thinking as epidemiology passed from the era of the germ theory into that of the search for causes of chronic noncontagious diseases. It was he who drew attention to the effect of specific context in that evolution. He recognized the influence of the microbiology laboratory on that early set of criteria for causality, the Henle–Koch postulates, as against the influence of human population studies on later criteria. He applied this thinking to his quest to discover causes both of infectious diseases (for example, the role of the Epstein–Barr virus in infectious mononucleosis) and of chronic diseases (for example, the role of the same virus in lymphomas). In short, Alfred Evans is well traveled in both the history and the practice of the subject of this book.

The territory is broad. The history is treated both generally, as criteria evolved, and specifically, as these criteria apply to a large array of diseases. I found much that was new to me in the accounts of the state of knowledge about the causes of many of these diseases and, equally, of the ways in which that knowledge was won. I recommend this book to students and researchers—which is to say all of us—in epidemiology, in clinical medicine, in microbiology and related fields. All should find the book instructive, always interesting, and frequently illuminating.

Mervyn Susser, M.D.
Gertrude H. Sergievsky Professor Emeritus
    and Special Lecturer
Columbia University
New York, New York

Preface

This monograph is a chronological account of the development of our concepts, postulates, and guidelines concerning disease causation, beginning with the postulates of Jacob Henle (1840) and of Robert Koch (1882, 1890). These Henle–Koch postulates have become the "golden rules" that have guided many investigators in establishing a relationship between a disease and a new etiological agent or risk factor. Some persons believe that if the postulates are fully met, then that risk factor is the cause of that disease, and if they are not met, it is not the cause. This historical review will emphasize that the postulates were directed only at bacterial diseases, that Koch himself felt they could not be fulfilled by many common bacterial diseases, and that fulfillment of only the first two postulates might be enough to establish causation.

Many other limitations to the postulates have appeared in the more than 100 years since their publication (Evans, 1977, 1980). The discovery of viruses has necessitated repeated modifications of these postulates, as have their applicability to immunological, chronic, and malignant diseases, and their use in law courts in cases of alleged occupational exposure. Changing technology and new concepts of pathogenesis, multiple causation, and the web of interacting factors have all required the introduction of new concepts of causation. Even the word "cause" has been replaced in chronic disease studies by "risk factors," and most infectious diseases require cofactors in their production. This book will review these chronological developments and show how various guidelines apply to various types of illness.

This book is not a methods book that outlines the laboratory and epidemiological studies that help establish causation. A recent book of which the present writer is co-author deals with methods in observational epidemiology, including both infectious and noninfectious diseases (Kelsey, Thompson, and Evans, 1986). Other recent texts on methodology that deal mainly with chronic disease, such as Hennekens and Buring (1986) and Rothman (1986), should also be consulted. Susser's excellent earlier book, *Causal Thinking in the Health Sciences* (1973), is recommended for a conceptual approach, and a recent book by Rothman (1986) reviews ways of establishing causal inferences from epidemiological data.

The questions of concept and theoretical methods to establish causation (if that is indeed possible) are not the subject of this book. This is a historical review, and the guidelines and postulates discussed are meant to be neither absolute nor unchanging but, rather, merely road maps to approaching practical levels of proof to guide prevention, intervention, and public policy. The reader will also find repetition in some of the chapters, such as those dealing with the clinical illness promotion factor (Chapter 11) and subclinical epidemiology (Chapter 12). This is done to make each chapter a coherent entity, so that a reader interested in a particular group of diseases or concepts can find a relatively complete discussion in a single chapter without the need to read the whole book.

The material presented here is, in part, derived from material already published in various articles by the author, but many new themes have been added. Finally, the author makes no claim for originality in these concepts. They are based on the work of others. My only hope is that the reader has some pleasure on this chronological journey and perhaps even gains a perspective on the ever-changing need for new concepts of causation and of risk factors in the pathogenesis of disease. The criteria of causation presented are meant to be practical guidelines to seeking evidence that differentiates causation and association. The reader interested in the basic rationale and philosophy of causal inferences should read the books and articles written or edited by Greenland and Morgenstern (1988), Rothman (1976, 1986), and Susser (1973, 1991). The recent article by Susser is an excellent brief summary of various viewpoints and provides a useful definition of terms (Susser, 1991).

References

Evans AS: Limitations to Koch's postulates. *Lancet* **2:**1277–1278, 1977.

Evans AS: Discussion, in Lilienfeld AM (ed): *Time, Places and Persons: Aspects of the History of Epidemiology.* Baltimore, Johns Hopkins University Press, 1980, pp. 94–98.

Greenland S, Morgenstern H: Classification schemes for epidemiologic research designs. *J Clin Epidemiol* **41:**715–716, 1988.

Henle J: *On Miasmata and Contagie.* Rosen G (trans). Baltimore, Johns Hopkins University Press, 1938.

Hennekens CA, Buring J: *Epidemiology in Medicine.* Boston, Little Brown & Co, 1987.

Kelsey J, Thompson WD, Evans AS: *Observational Epidemiology.* London, Oxford University Press, 1986.

Koch R: Die Aetiologie der Tuberkulose. *Berl Klin Wochenschr* **15:**428–448, 1882.

Koch R: Ueber bacteriologische Forschung, in *Verh X Int Med Congr Berlin, 1890,* 1892, p 35.

Rothman KJ: Causes. *Am J Epidemiol* **104:**587–592, 1976.

Rothman KJ: *Modern Epidemiology*. Boston, Little Brown & Co, 1986.

Susser M: *Causal Thinking in the Health Sciences: Concepts and Strategies*. London, Oxford University Press, 1973.

Susser M: What is a cause and how do we know one? A grammar of pragmatic epidemiology. *Am J Epidemiol* **133:**635–648, 1991.

Contents

Concepts and Background of Causation

Causality in the Natural Sciences

Since the beginning of history, natural science has been based on common experience. Primitive man observed things in space and in time and made conjectures for the explanation of natural phenomena (Lenzen, 1954). Such experiences led to the belief that the sun is the cause of light, that fire caused smoke, and that injury caused pain. They led to the concept that causation is a process by which one phenomenon, the cause, gives rise to another phenomenon, the effect.

Our understanding of this relationship involves a continuity between primitive experience and natural phenomena. In his book *Causality in Natural Science,* Lenzen (1954) discusses two types of causality—one he calls dynamical causality, in which the same cause is succeeded by the same effect, and the other he calls statistical causality, in which the same cause is followed by a distributed effect. In human diseases, the former represents a one-on-one relationship between a specific cause and a given disease from which our early concepts of the causation of infectious diseases arose. The latter expresses the concept of the biological spectrum, in which a single cause can result in a spectrum of clinical syndromes. To these concepts was later added the observation that the same effect, or in this case, clinical syndromes, could result from several different causes. In clinical diseases in both man and animals, either the cause or the effect could change, depending on the nature of the causative agent, the environment in which it operates, and the characteristics of the involved host (animal or human) in terms of age, genetic disposition, and the existence of other diseases at the time the cause is operative (Evans, 1976).

This book will deal largely with the way that various guidelines for establishing a causal relationship between a cause or causes and a disease or clinical syndrome emerged chronologically. It will discuss how these guidelines had to be modified to keep up with the development of new techniques of identifying the cause and of new concepts of the pathogenesis (particularly the mechanism by which disease results after exposure, and the various host factors involved in this interaction). The conceptual approaches and methodology are well described in Susser's excellent book, *Causal Thinking in the Health Sciences* (Susser, 1973).

Concepts of Contagion

The concept of contagion, or the direct spread of infectious diseases by contact, appears to have existed during early human history, as evidenced by references to leprosy recorded in the Bible (Leviticus, Chapters XII and XIV). The first formulation of the concept of contagion is attributed by many authors (Garrison, 1966; Bulloch, 1938; Ackernecht, 1982; Spink, 1978) to Girolamo Fracastoro (or Hieronymus Fracastorius in the Latinized form) in 1546. Fracastoro was a physician, scholar, poet, physicist, geologist, astrologist, and thinker. He was born in Verona, Italy about 1478 and died in 1553. He attended the University of Padua and is known for his Latin poem, *Syphilis sive morbus Gallicus,* or "The Sinister Sheperd," from which we derive the term "syphilis" for the venereal disease.

Fracastoro's work on contagion (1930) was written in Latin and consists of 77 pages in a condensed style not easy to translate or interpret. Indeed, much controversy has arisen over the various meanings read into it by different historians. It comprises three books of which the first and most important deals with the theory of contagion, the second with an account of several contagious diseases, and the third with their cure. In the first chapter, contagion is defined as an infection that passes from one individual to another and is different from the corruption in milk or meat. Contagion is present in three different forms: (1) contagion by contact alone, (2) contagion by fomites, and (3) contagion at a distance. Fracastoro is quoted as saying of fomites, "I call fomites clothes, wooden things and other things of that sort which in themselves are not corrupted but are able to preserve the original germs of the contagion and to give rise to its transference to others" (Bulloch, 1938). He spoke of the "seminaria" of disease, which has been interpreted by some as referring to the "seeds" or "germs" of disease. But we must remember that he knew nothing about germs as we know them today, and that too much may have been read into his book and into its interpretation by some historians.

Howard-Jones is one exception and states that the claims for both Fracastoro and Jacob Henle (whom we will deal with in the next chapter) with respect to the theory of communicable diseases, are "unrealistic and grossly exaggerated" (Howard-Jones, 1973). He states that "these claims are based on selective quotations, translations of terms that never corresponded to any objective reality, by words that now refer to observed phenomena, and the application of hindsight to interpret in the language of experimental science what were only vague, and often manifestly incorrect, speculations."

I will not attempt to evaluate these criticisms in this book and will, in general, follow the interpretations of more traditional and less critical historians. In the 17th century, and prior to Henle in 1840, several concepts of contagion were presented. One of these was that of Thomas Sydenham (1624–1689), on theories of the genesis of epidemic diseases. Sydenham believed that each disease had a natural course of its own, and he wrote detailed descriptions of smallpox, continued and remittent fevers, pneumonia, rheumatism, erysipelas, quinsy, and St. Vitus dance (Spink, 1978). Richard Mead wrote a discourse on pestilential contagion, and James Lind, in the latter half of the 18th century, used the terms "infection" and "contagion" synonymously to cover all fevers of whatever kind that are imparted from one person to another (Howard-Jones, 1977). In 1831, Sir Gilbert Blane used the term "communicable," presumably for the first time, to avoid the epithets "contagious" and "infectious." The concept of an animate contagion and also of its specificity is attributed by Howard-Jones (1977) to Moreau de Jonnes in France in 1831 when the latter advised the Higher Council of Health that cholera was "incontestably" contagious and was a *"principle sui generis,* a germ . . . that possesses the power to develop and reproduce in the manner of organized beings, and which propagates itself by mediate or intermediate transmission from a sick to a healthy individual." In that same year, Hahnemann, the founder of homeopathy, published an appeal to "thinking friends of humanity," in which he maintained that cholera was transmitted by a "miasm probably consisting of innumerable invisible living organisms" that had the power of reproduction.

Epidemiology and Causation

Long before bacteria were discovered, epidemiological techniques were used to establish the cause and/or method of transmission of epidemics of both infectious and noninfectious diseases. If one can identify the source of the factor resulting in the disease or in its means of transmission through the environment, the disease may be prevented without actually characterizing or isolating the true causal agent. Similarly, the identification of a cofactor, or second risk factor, and its modification may also result in the control of the disease without knowledge of the exact causative agent. The guidelines for establishing causation of an agent in an epidemic were not often stated. An agent was usually thought to be causally related when its source or its method of transmission were interrupted and the epidemic ceased. Since epidemics may cease for several other reasons, such as the exhaustion or removal of susceptible persons, the idea of a cause-and-effect relationship was not always correct. As an example, the removal of the handle of the pump on Broad Street, as described in the classic study of cholera in London by John Snow in 1849, actually took place *after* the epidemic was on the wane. I will now present a number of other classic epidemiological studies and discuss the basis for presuming a causal relationship, before proceeding with the chronological development of criteria associating a specific cause with a given disease in *an individual*.

Causation of Epidemics in the Prebacteriology Era

Scurvy

In 1757, James Lind, a physician to the English Navy, published his investigations of outbreaks of scurvy among sailors on long voyages (Lind, 1953). His hypothesis of causation was that something was missing in the diet. He experimented by adding various dietary supplements to see if any of these were the cause, that is, if any would prevent or cure the condition. The test was carried out on the ship *Salisbury* in May 1747, on twelve subjects divided into groups of two, each given a different supplement to a common diet for six days. The diet included a quart of cider daily, elixir vitriol three times a day, two spoonfuls of vinegar daily, half a pint of sea water daily, two oranges and one lemon daily, and nutmeg three times a day. Lind stated the results as follows: "The consequences were that the most sudden and visible good effects were perceived from the use of oranges and lemons; one of those who had taken them being fit for duty."

From these replacement experiments, Lind deduced that a deficiency of citrus fruits was responsible, and that an appropriate supplement would provide a means of prevention as well as therapy. The British Navy eventually accepted this suggestion and, from 1795 on, required the inclusion of lime or lime juice in the diet on ships, hence the term "limey" for English sailors. While Lind's sample size seems very meager by modern standards, he did draw the right conclusions from it and showed that a disease could be due to the lack of something or the presence of something. Some 150 years later, Goldberger showed that another disease, pellagra, was a deficiency disease in a series of careful epidemiological studies carried out from 1914 to 1930 (Terris, 1964).

Lead Colic

An outbreak of a disease characterized by abdominal pain and cramps and termed "the epidemic colic" occurred in Devonshire, England beginning in

1724. In 1767, George Baker, a practitioner and physician to Her Majesty's household, investigated the possible cause. His investigations suggested that drinking cider could be the cause, but he found that persons drinking cider in counties other than Devon had little colic. This led him to suspect the presence of "some fraudulent or accidental adulterant" in the cider from Devonshire. By examining hospital records, he found that Devon patients outnumbered those from Hereford, Glouster, and Worcester counties by a ratio of 8:1. On examining the possible reasons for this, he found that no lead was used in any part of the cider-making process in Herefordshire. In Devon, however, exposure to lead was possible in several steps, including grinding, pressing, and even storing in casks to prevent souring. His own testing confirmed that Devon cider contained lead, and this was further confirmed by a chemist.

In this study, Baker established the cause through epidemiological differences between two groups, one exposed to lead in cider and the other, not so exposed. He then confirmed his epidemiological evidence by an actual demonstration of the lead content in Devon cider in two separate laboratories. On the basis of these findings, he alerted Devon residents to the dangers of lead in cider by distributing copies of his essay, thus applying his epidemiological findings to prevention.

Cholera

John Snow (1813–1858), a London anesthesiologist who administered chloroform to Queen Victoria during childbirth and was a pioneer in this field, also carried out classic epidemiological studies on cholera. He used two techniques. In the first, he investigated an outbreak of cholera on Broad Street in London in 1849. He suspected the Broad Street pump as the source, and water as the vehicle of transmission. While he did not compare the illness rates between those who drank and those who did not drink the water in the first study, he had other bases of comparison. He noted that workers in a nearby brewery who got their water from their own source did not develop cholera, that certain individuals who were away did not fall ill, and that anyone from another vicinity who was supplied with well water from the pump came down with cholera. From these observations, he concluded that something carried in the water resulted in cholera among those who drank it, and he advised the town fathers to remove the handle from the pump to control the outbreak. After this was done, the epidemic ceased (Snow, 1936). This idea, however, was criticized by students of epidemiology who carefully conducted their own studies on the outbreak. They knew that the epidemic was actually on the wane by the time that the handle of the pump was removed. This criticism was also made by Max von Pettenkofer, the great German hygienist, who did not believe that cholera was transmitted directly by water but first had to acquire some virulence factor by passage through soil (the so-called Boden theory). His views were expressed in a book published in 1855, and his critique of Snow appeared in a series of articles published in *The Lancet* in 1884 (Pettenkofer, 1884). Snow's initial findings were not accepted by the medical council, which appointed a committee to reexamine the evidence. Snow was later made a member of the commission. In a case-control study of those exposed and not exposed to the well water, it was clear that cholera developed much more often in those exposed (3,790 versus 940).

The second of Snow's studies was much more convincing, although not without some objections from Pettenkofer and others. This was a retrospective cohort study of cholera deaths occurring in households supplied in parallel by water from one of two water companies. Both had derived water from the Thames River at points heavily polluted with sewage. However, between 1849 and 1854 the Lambeth Company relocated its source to a less contaminated site. When the cholera epidemic occurred in 1854, about two thirds of London's population was being served by one company or the other. Snow determined the number of houses supplied by each and calculated the cholera death rate per 10,000 houses for the first several weeks. The rates among persons supplied by the two companies were then compared with each other and with the rest of London. The results are given in Table 1.1. The analysis indicated that the Southwark and Vauxhall Company had cholera death rates of 315 per 10,000 homes, which was 8.5 times higher than the Lambeth Company's 37 per 10,000 and 5.3 times higher than the 59 per 10,000 recorded for the rest of London. It is noteworthy that Snow employed what might be called matched controls, as represented by the houses within the same neighborhoods, as well as a general population control, represented by the rest of the houses in London. From these and other observations, Snow inferred the existence of a "cholera poison" transmitted by polluted water. This prompted the passage of legislation that, by 1857, all water companies should be filtering their water.

Another contributor to the epidemiology of cholera was William Budd

Table 1.1

Deaths from Cholera per 10,000 Houses by Source of Water Supply, London, 1854[a]

Water supply	Number of houses	Deaths from cholera	Deaths per 10,000 houses
Southwark and Vauxhall Co.	40,046	1263	315
Lambeth Co.	26,107	98	37
Rest of London	256,423	1422	59

[a]From Snow (1936).

(1811–1880), who also proposed the water-borne nature of typhoid fever. In a pamphlet published in 1849, the year of Snow's first publication, Budd said that he confirmed observations made by a Mr. Brittan and a Mr. Swayne of the presence of organisms in the "rice water" stool of cholera patients and that he found them in almost every specimen of water from cholera districts, but not in water from "healthy quarters" (Budd, 1849a). It was not quite clear what he observed, although there were drawings of them, and he called them fungi. His deductions, however, were certainly accurate:

1. The cause of malignant cholera is a living organism of distinct species.
2. This organism—in shapes hereafter to be described—is taken by the act of swallowing into the intestinal canal, and there becomes infinitely multiplied by the self-propagation that is characteristic of living beings.
3. The presence and propagation of these organisms in the intestinal canal and the action they exert there are the causes of the peculiar flux that is characteristic of malignant cholera, and that, taken with its consequences, immediate and remote, constitutes the disease.
4. The new organisms are developed only in the human intestine.
5. These organisms are disseminated to society in the following ways:
   • in the air, in the form of impalpable or palpable particles
   • in contact with articles of food
   • and principally, in the drinking water of infected places (Budd, 1849b).

These observations were fully confirmed, except for the airborne aspect, when the organism was more fully identified. This was done in 1854 by Pacini, who found the organism in the intestinal tract, named the organism *Vibrio cholerae*, and incriminated it as the causative agent of cholera (Howard-Jones, 1971). Despite these earlier observations, Robert Koch is generally hailed as the discoverer of the organism (1884). He grew it in bacterial culture from cases of cholera in Egypt and India (Koch, 1893). While the earlier observations on the cause of cholera did not meet the postulates proposed by Koch for establishing proof of causation, including Koch's own findings, they certainly pointed to the presence of some organism in cholera stools that was transmitted by drinking water, and these observations were the basis for successful prevention. Thus, proof of causality may not always require demonstration of the presence of the organism for successful control.

Puerperal Sepsis

One last example of epidemiological techniques and their applications in the prevention of disease without actually culturing or identifying the presumed causative agent itself is the work of Ignaz Semmelweis (1818–1865) on puerperal sepsis or childbed fever, as it was popularly known. His basic observations were made in 1846 in a hospital in Vienna called the Allgemeines Krankenhaus. He noted the high mortality rate of 11% from childbed fever among women being delivered by physicians on Obstetrical Ward Division 1, as compared with only 3.38% among women being delivered by midwives on Division 2. Semmelweis was working on Division 1 and often conducted, with his students, autopsies on women who had died of puerperal sepsis prior to coming to the obstetrical ward. One of his associates, Kolletschka, had developed lesions similar to those of childbed fever, after receiving a stab wound while dissecting a cadaver in the anatomy laboratory. Kolletschka subsequently died. Semmelweis believed that the same substance that had killed Kolletschka was being carried by physicians from the dead house to the lying-in ward, and this explained the higher mortality rate on Division 1. The mortality on Division 2 was lower because the midwives were not involved in autopsy work.

This made up his hypothesis of causation and spread. To prove it, he obtained a decree in 1847 that no student attending on his ward could at the same time attend on postmortem examinations. Students who want to do both should scrub their hands in a solution of chloride of lime before examining patients on his obstetrical ward. Within 7 months, the epidemic had practically stopped, and the mortality subsequently dropped from 11.4 to 1.27% (Semmelweis, 1981). His observations were strengthened statistically over the next 14 years, when the mortality from childbed fever remained at a low 3.34% among 56,104 women delivered on the physicians' ward, as compared with 2.8% on the midwives' ward. Thus, by a case–control study he had established a difference in mortality between the two wards, by observation and deduction had formulated a hypothesis of the origin and spread of the causative agent, and by breaking the chain of transmission had markedly reduced the incidence of the disease. While these facts may seem convincing to us as proof of causation, they were not accepted by his colleagues or his chief. Perhaps this is because to our mind they make bacteriological sense, whereas to his colleagues they did not, as the age of bacteriology did not begin until some 40 years later with the work of Pasteur and Koch.

The Age of Bacteriological Discovery

The brief sketch of the major discoveries in microbiology given here is derived from Bulloch (1938), Spink (1978), and Ackernecht (1982). The reader is referred to them for more details. The contributions of Henle, Klebs, and Koch will be the main focus of the next chapter because they are relevant to the development of Koch's famous postulates of causation.

Table 1.2 lists some of the major discoveries in microbiology over a period of about 50 years. Most of the earlier observations were isolated and practical ones that preceded the great discoveries of Pasteur and later, of Koch. One of the earliest contributions was made in 1835 by a lawyer named Agostino Bassi. He

Table 1.2
Some Early Discoveries in Bacteriology, 1835–1889[a]

Year	Disease	Cause	Discoverer
1835	Diseases of silkworm	Fungi	Bassi
1837	Vaginal infections	*Trichomonas vaginalis*	Donne
1844	Skin diseases	Fungi	Gruby
1850	Anthrax in animals	Anthrax bacillus	Davaine, Rayer
1854	Cholera	*Vibrio cholerae*	Pacini
1855	Anthrax in animals	Anthrax bacillus	Pollender
1860	Trichinosis	Trichinae	Virchow, Zender
1862	"Diseases" of wine	Bacteria	Pasteur
1865	Diseases of silkworms	Bacteria	Pasteur
1868	Relapsing fever	Spirilla	Obermeier
1872	Septicemia	Bacteria	Coze, Feltz, Davaine
1876	Anthrax	Anthrax bacillus	Koch
1878	Wound infection	Bacteria	Koch
1879	Gonorrhea	Bacillus	Neisser
1880	Typhoid fever	Bacillus	Eberth, Gaffky
	Leprosy	Bacillus	Hansen
	Malaria	Parasite	Laveran
1882	Tuberculosis	Tubercle bacillus	Koch
	Glanders	Bacillus	Löffler
1883	Cholera	Bacillus	Koch
	Erysipelas	Bacillus	Fehleisen
1884	Diphtheria	Bacillus	Klebs, Löffler
	Tetanus	Bacillus	Nikolaier, Kitasato
	Pneumonia	Bacillus	Fraenkel
1887	Epidemic meningitis	Bacillus	Weichselbaum
	Malta fever	Bacillus	Bruce
1889	Soft chancre	Bacillus	Ducrey

[a]Adapted from Ackernecht (1982).

demonstrated that certain diseases of the silkworm were contagious, being produced by fungi, and from this he drew conclusions with far-reaching implications on contagious diseases in general, including variola, typhus, plague, syphilis, wound gangrene, and cholera (Bulloch, 1938; Ackerneckt, 1982). Indeed, Bulloch (1938) states, "It is impossible to read the works of Bassi without realizing that he was a pioneer . . . and that he was the founder of the doctrine of parasitic microbes and precursor of Schwann, Pasteur, and Koch." Donne described *Trichomonas vaginalis* in 1837; Schoenlein described the fungus of favus in 1839, and Gruby, other fungi causing skin disease in 1844.

In 1850, bacteria were added to the list of pathogenic microorganisms, when Davaine (1812–1882) and Rayer (1793–1867) discovered the anthrax bacillus in the blood of animals dying from the disease, and succeeded in transmitting it to other animals. Pollender published the same findings in 1855 based on work he had done earlier, in 1849. The large size of the anthrax bacillus made it a likely candidate for early detection under the microscope. The concept of spread by contagion was supported by transmission experiments such as those performed by Rayer on glanders in 1837, by Klencke on tuberculosis in 1843 (for which he did not receive recognition), and by Villemin in 1865 (Ackernecht, 1982).

The development of the new science of microbiology was due largely to the genius of Louis Pasteur (1822–1895), the son of a tanner in Dole in the Jura mountains of France. He was educated as a chemist and later held professorships in physics at the Lycée of Dijon in 1848, and in chemistry in Strasbourg in 1852. In 1857 he went to Paris as the director of scientific studies in the École Normale. His early discoveries were in the field of chemistry, where he demonstrated the existence of molecular dyssymmetry. Through his studies on fermentation in 1857, he showed conclusively that molecular dyssymmetry was the result of the growth of various microorganisms. In a series of brilliant experiments in 1862, Pasteur eliminated the theory of spontaneous generation of bacteria. In 1863 he saved the wine industry in France by the process now termed "pasteurization." His studies were extended in 1877 to the causes and prevention of diseases in humans and animals. His many contributions in this area include the discovery of the protective properties of attenuated organisms in inducing immunity against several diseases, particularly fowl cholera (in 1880), anthrax (in 1881), swine erysipelas (in 1882) and rabies (in 1884) (Bulloch, 1938). In his honor, the Pasteur Institute was established in Paris in 1888.

The discoveries of Pasteur and other bacteriologists provided the basis for the formulation of concepts of causation. They were not, however, formally recognized as such at that time, even though the strongest evidence of a causal relationship between a suspected causal agent and any infectious disease is perhaps Pasteur's demonstration that the organisms he had isolated from a certain disease could be used in attenuated form to prevent that disease.

References

Ackernecht EH: *A Short History of Medicine*. Baltimore, Johns Hopkins University Press, 1982.

Baker G: *An Essay Concerning the Cause of the Endemic Colic of Devonshire*. London, Delta Omega Society, 1958.

Budd W: Alleged discovery of the cause of cholera. *Lancet* **2:**371–372, 1849a.

Budd W: *Malignant Cholera: Its Modes and Propagation and Its Prevention*. London, Churchill, 1849b.

Bulloch W: *The History of Bacteriology*. London, Oxford University Press, 1938.

Evans AS: Causation and disease: The Henle–Koch postulates revisited. *Yale J Biol Med* **49:**175–195, 1976.

Evans AS: Two errors in enteric epidemiology. The stories of Austin Flint and Max von Pettenkofer. *Rev Infect Dis* **7:**434–440, 1985.

Fracastoro G: *De Contagrone et Contagrosis Morbis et Earum Curatione*, Libri III, Wright WC (trans). London, GP Putnam's Sons, 1930.

Garrison FH: *Contributions to the History of Medicine*. New York, Hafner, 1966.

Howard-Jones N: Choleranomolies: The unhistory of medicine as exemplified by cholera. *Perspect Biol Med* **13:**422–433, 1971.

Howard-Jones N: Gelsenkirchen typhoid outbreak of 1901. Robert Koch and the dead hand of Max von Pettenkofer. *Br Med J* **1:**103–105, 1973.

Howard-Jones N: Fracastoro and Henle: A reappraisal of their contributions to the concept of communicable disease. *Med Hist* **21:**61–68, 1977.

Koch R: Ueber die Cholerabakterien. *Deutsch Med Wochenschr* **10:**725–728, 1884.

Koch R: Uber den augenblicklichen Stand der bakteriolischen Cholera Diagnose. *J Hyg Infektionskr* **14:**319–426, 1893.

Lenzen VF: *Causality in Natural Science*. Springfield, Ill, Charles C Thomas Publisher, 1954.

Lind J: *Treatise on Scurvy*, Stewart CP, Guthrie D (eds). Edinburgh, Edinburgh University Press, 1953.

Pettenkofer M: Cholera. *Lancet* **2:**769–771, 816–819, 861–864, 904–905, 992–994, 1042–1043, 1086–1088, 1884.

Semmelweiss IP: The etiology of childbed fever (English translation), in *Kelley's Classics,* vol. V, 1981, p 338.

Snow J: On the mode of communication of cholera, in *Snow on Cholera*. New York, The Commonwealth Fund, 1936, pp 1–175.

Spink WW: *Infectious Disease Prevention in the Nineteenth and Twentieth Centuries*. Minneapolis, University of Minneapolis Press, 1978.

Susser M: *Causal Thinking in the Health Sciences: Concepts and Strategies*. London, Oxford University Press, 1978.

Terris M: *Goldberger on Pellagra*. Baton Rouge, Louisiana University Press, 1964.

Causation and Bacterial Diseases

While the first postulates of causation are generally attributed to Robert Koch, his contributions, like most advances in science, rest on the work of others who preceded him, especially that of his teacher, Jakob Henle, and another great German bacteriologist, Edwin Klebs. The work of these three men will be reviewed in this chapter, and the applicability of the Koch postulates to several bacterial diseases will be discussed, including the pathogens of Legionnaire's disease and Lyme disease.

Jacob Henle

Many authors attribute the first enunciation of the criteria for causation in bacterial diseases to Jacob Henle (Figure 2.1) in 1840, some 40 years before Koch's contributions to bacteriology, and before methods for bacterial culture and isolation were known. Henle was born in Fürth, Bavaria, Germany in 1809 and died in 1885. He was educated in Bonn and Heidelberg and was a student of Johannes Müller, whom he followed to Berlin. He became a professor of anatomy in Zurich at the age of 31. As anatomist and pathologist, he made many contributions to and wrote textbooks on medical science, as summarized in Table 2.1.

His contributions to causation comprise the first 82 pages of his *Pathologische Untersuchungen* entitled *"Von den Miasmen und Contagien und von den miasmatisch-contagiosen Krankheiten"* (Henle, 1840). It has been translated into English by the historian Rosen (Henle, 1938) and discussed extensively by Bulloch (1938) in his book *The History of Bacteriology*. Henle's essay is a theoretical one and does not involve original contributions by Henle himself. Indeed, Henle states it contains "few facts and many reflections." The main object was to establish the hypothesis that "the material and contagion is not only organic but living, endowed with individual life and standing to the diseased

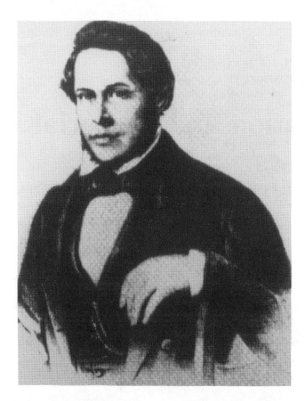

Figure 2.1.   Jacob Henle, 1809–1885 (reprinted from Evans, 1976, with permission).

body in the relation of a parasitic organism." He discussed three types of epidemic diseases: (1) miasmatas, alone, such as ague; (2) miasmatic-contagious diseases, such as the exanthemata, cholera, plague, and influenza; and (3) contagious diseases, such as syphilis, itch, rabies, and probably glanders and foot-and-mouth diseases. He thought that the discharges from the body contained the material of infection and that the contagia must be living. Disease does not break out all at once for there was, Henle felt, a *stadium latentis* in which the contagion is increasing, and when the necessary increase is achieved the effect on the body is fever and inflammation. We would call this the incubation period of the disease. He foresaw the difficulties of obtaining proof that his views were correct, and that even if some agent were identified in a disease, it might be purely accidental and have no causal relation to the disease itself. Of utmost importance was his statement:

> Before microscopic forms can be regarded as the cause of contagion in man, they must be constantly found in contagious material. They must be isolated from it and their strength tested.

Table 2.1
Contributions of Jacob Henle

Eye:	Histology of Retina
	Physiology of lachrymal canal
	Construction and development of fibers of crystalline lens
Larynx:	Evolution and development
Kidney:	Henle's ampulla, canal, cells, fibrin, sphincter, tubule
Books:	*Handbook of Systemic Anatomy*
	Handbook of General Anatomy
	Handbook of Rational Pathology

Bulloch (1938) states, "This constant presence, isolation, and testing of the isolated object is the unassailable basis on which all the subsequent work on pathogenic bacteria has been built up, and Henle's statement of the proposition contains all the elements habitually referred to as the 'postulates of Koch.' " Many other historians seem to agree with this general assessment. Indeed, Castiglione (1947) and Rosen (Henle, 1938), for example, as well as this author, have suggested renaming the postulates "the Henle–Koch postulates" (Evans, 1976). However, others such as Howard-Jones (1977), Doetsch (1982), and Carter (1982) disagree with this view and feel that Henle deserves little or no credit for Koch's postulates. Howard-Jones is particularly strong on the subject, as well as critical of the contributions of Fracastoro, described in the previous chapter. He states that "The speculations of both Fracastoro and Henle have been the object of an immoderate and uncritical adulation that is entirely unmerited" (Howard-Jones, 1977).

Whatever the truth of the matter is, and one may be tempted to read too much into early findings, it is clear that Henle eventually got to the University of Göttingen, where Robert Koch studied medicine and became his student. However, it is also true that Koch did not mention Henle in the statement of his postulates in the key papers of 1882 and 1890 (Koch, 1882a, 1890). Koch did refer to the contributions to causality of another German scientist, Edwin Klebs, in his 1878 paper on wound infections (as quoted by Carter, 1982), and in his second 1882 paper on tuberculosis (Koch, 1882b).

Edwin Klebs

Klebs was born in 1834 in Königsberg, Germany and died in 1913. A fine summary of his life and contributions was written by Baumgartner (1935) in honor of the 100th anniversary of his birth, from which much of this discussion is derived.* He studied medicine at Würzburg under a stimulating faculty that included Virchow and Kölliker. Virchow impressed him so deeply that he followed Virchow to Berlin in 1861, three years after the latter's *Cellularpathologie* had appeared. After Berlin, Klebs worked in many universities, including Bern (1866), Würzburg (1872), Prague (1873), and Zurich (1882). He then went to Karlsruhe for a year, after which he came to America. He first settled in a private tuberculosis sanatorium in Ashville, North Carolina; then in 1896, he moved to Chicago to become professor of pathology at Rush Medical College.

In 1900 he returned to Europe. His many contributions to bacteriology are given in Table 2.2. These include a treatise on anthrax, which appeared a year after Koch's work; the first descriptions of the bacillus of typhoid fever and of diphtheria; and extended studies on cholera and malaria. He described the use of solid media for bacterial cultures using sturgeon's glue in 1872, three years before Koch did. However, unlike Koch, he used this technique in studying different stages in the growth of the same organism, rather than as a means of separating bacterial species. His contributions to the concepts of causation are included in a paper on tuberculosis published in 1877 (Klebs, 1877), five years before Koch's postulates on the causal proof of the tubercle in tuberculosis (Koch, 1882a).

The following excerpts are from Baumgartner (1935), who also includes the original German version of the relevant parts of Klebs's remarks on causation. [Carter (1982) also emphasizes Klebs's contribution to causation prior to Koch, and provides an English translation from another 1877 paper by Klebs.] Klebs discussed the anatomy of the local lesion in tuberculosis and then made the following remarks:

> The simplest way to prove that the cells of the diseased animal neither produce nor in any way increase the virus of tuberculosis is to cultivate it outside of the organism, under conditions which do not destroy the life processes of the cells of the warm-blooded hosts. If, under such conditions, there is still an increase in the main action, this must be dependent upon the presence of tissues of the animal body, remains of dead tissue cells, or upon components of the inoculum which, usually foreign to the animal, developed within the tubercle.

Klebs then described the use of egg whites as a culture medium, and continued:

> If it can thus be established, as the older inoculation experiments indicated and the ones presented today corroborate, that tuberculosis infection can not only be induced by inoculation of tuberculous tissues but also with organisms which are found in such tissues and can be grown outside the body, it becomes necessary to establish the presence of these organisms in the diseased tissues from human and animal tuberculosis.

---

*I was not earlier aware of Baumgartner's paper (Evans, 1976).

Table 2.2
Contributions of Edwin Klebs and Robert Koch[a]

Year	Klebs	Koch
1872	Bacteriology of gunshot wounds Use of solid culture media	
1873	Produced tuberculosis in animals by injecting milk from infected cows	
1876		Treatise on cause of anthrax
1877	Treatise on cause of anthrax Studies on tuberculosis Postulated of causation	
1878	Inoculated primates with organism of syphilis	Studies of septic infection of animals
1880	Description of typhoid bacillus	
1881		Introduction of solid culture media
1882		Treatise on etiology of tuberculosis The postulates
1883	Description of diphtheria organism	
1884	Studies on cholera	Isolated cause of Asiatic cholera
1885	Worked on etiology of cholera	
1889	Studies on malaria	
1890		Tuberculin discovered
1891		Human and bovine TB are different
1892	Pathology and treatment of cholera	
1893		Studies on Rhodesian red water fever, recurring fever, trypanosomiasis
1896		Investigates rinderpest, sleeping sickness
1905		Awarded Nobel Prize
1908	Use of attenuated TB organism to produce immunity in guinea pigs and humans	

[a]From Baumgartner (1935) and Bulloch (1938).

To prove the above, he described at length the organisms he had seen in the tubercles. The final step in proving causation is stated concisely:

> Small amounts of the products of this cultivation experiment inoculated into the peritoneum of healthy animals, result in the development of a miliary tuberculosis exactly as does the implantation of tuberculous tissue in the same locus.

Little comment was apparently aroused over these experimental results at the time of publication for, as Baumgartner (1935) points out, ". . it is evident that they include the salient points of the well-known Koch postulates upon which the recognition of any organism as the etiological agent of a given clinical entity has subsequently been based."

Klebs was interested in tuberculosis throughout his entire scientific life. In addition to the reproduction of the disease in animals, using milk from infected cows, he described the use of attenuated strains of tubercle bacilli from cold-blooded animals in the development of active immunity in guinea pigs and humans (Klebs, 1908).

Robert Koch

Inseparably linked with Pasteur in the creation of the science of bacteriology is the name of Robert Koch (Figure 2.2). He was born in 1843 in Clausthal, Hannover, Germany, the son of a mining engineer. He studied medicine at the University of Göttingen under Wöhler, Meissner, and Henle. His arrival in Göttingen to study medicine is rather humorously depicted in a sketch (Figure 2.3) from Knight's popular biography (Knight, 1961). In the sketch, a local dachshund regards Koch suspiciously, and Koch appears to be looking at the Löwenbrau beer sign, as though finding it inviting. In reality, Koch probably spent little time in taverns, for he was a serious student. Later in life, though, he did enjoy his beer.

At Göttingen, it is said that it was Jacob Henle, the professor of anatomy, who aroused Koch's interest in the study of very small organisms. Henle also offered a prize to the medical student who in 10 months' time could solve a then unanswered anatomical problem. Koch won first prize and received 80 talers (about 60 dollars), which permitted him to return for another semester without asking his father for tuition money (Knight, 1961). As a result of winning the prize, he was also made a full-fledged assistant in the Museum of Pathology at the age of 22. He graduated with honors in 1866, after which he went to Berlin as an intern in the Charity Hospital. There, he attended lectures given by the famous pathologist, Rudolf Virchow. He later passed the state medical examination and accepted an offer of an assistantship at the General Hospital in Hamburg. It was there that he had an opportunity to study cholera patients in an outbreak of the

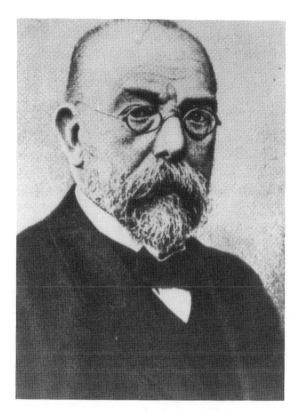

Figure 2.2.   Robert Koch, 1843–1910 (reprinted from Evans, 1976, with permission).

disease in 1866. It is said that he observed the organism under his microscope and made drawings of it, although not recognizing the significance of what he saw.

He moved to Langenhagen at the end of 1866 to work as resident physician in a hospital for the mentally ill. In 1867, he married Emmy Fraatz, who was from his hometown. After 2 years at Langenhagen, he left to practice medicine at Niemegk and then at Rakwitz. In 1869, Koch entered military service as a volunteer surgeon during the Franco-Prussian War, during which three of his brothers died. After his return to Rakwitz at the request of the town, he applied and was accepted for the job of District Physician for the whole area around Wollstein, a small Posen town near Rakwitz. It was during his 8 years there that he began his serious work in bacteriology, despite the heavy demands of being a country practitioner.

Koch isolated the anthrax organism from the blood of ill sheep in his home laboratory in Wollstein (Koch, 1910, 1938). He showed the organism to be ab-

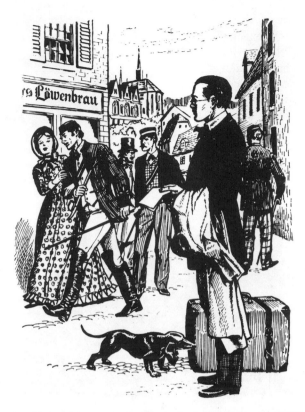

Figure 2.3. Robert Koch arriving to attend medical school at the University of Göttingen (reprinted from Knight, 1961).

sent from the blood of healthy sheep, and demonstrated the growth of the organisms in "hanging drops." Koch supported Pasteur's concept that every disease might be caused by a specific germ. In 1876, at age 32, Koch presented his findings and demonstrated his laboratory techniques on anthrax to members of the Botanical Institute in Breslau (Koch, 1876); among those present were Leopold Auerbach, the physiologist; Julius Cohnheim, the pathologist; and Carl Weigert, who was the first to stain cultures with dyes. The demonstration lasted three days. His audience, especially Cohnheim, was enthusiastic and delighted over the findings. Koch had emphasized that "each disease is caused by one particular microbe—and by one alone. Only an anthrax microbe causes anthrax; only a typhoid microbe can cause typhoid fever."

On Cohnheim's urging, Koch submitted his findings to Rudolf Virchow, the greatest name in German medical science at the time, and went to visit him in Berlin. Virchow, however, was not impressed or interested in Koch's discovery, and Koch left, bitter and disappointed. He returned to his country practice at

Wollstein, but did eventually publish his findings (Koch, 1876) and continued his association with Cohnheim's laboratory in Breslau. In 1880, Koch went to work at the Imperial Health Office in Berlin. There, he developed a solid medium for the culture of bacteria and began his work on tuberculosis, collaborating with Friedrich Löffler and George Gaffky. On March 24, 1882, he was able to announce before the Berlin Physiological Society his discovery of the isolation of the tubercle bacillus and to present evidence that it caused the human disease, tuberculosis (Koch, 1882a, 1932). His audience included Dr. Bois-Reymond, von Helmholtz, Ehrlich, von Behring, Cohnheim, and "the professor of professors," Rudolf Virchow. Koch's presentation and evidence were so complete that all were convinced, and no one, even Virchow, had any questions or comments. A sketch from Knight (1961) portrays the presentation (Figure 2.4). Paul Ehrlich wrote later: "That evening was engraved in my memory as the most

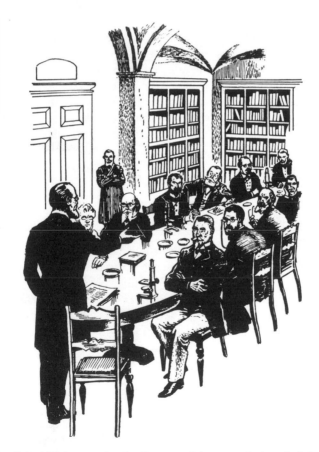

Figure 2.4. Robert Koch presenting the discovery of the cause of tuberculosis before the Berlin Physiological Society, March 28, 1882 (from Knight, 1961).

majestic event I have ever participated in." Similarly, Löffler is reported to have
said afterwards that "There was no one in the room who heard him who could be
anything else but convinced that he had made an epoch-making discovery."
Koch's findings were published in 1882 in his classic paper "Die Atiologie der
Tuberkulose" (Koch, 1882a).

The news of Koch's discovery spread with great rapidity, considering the
limited speed of communication at that time. Indeed, investigators today would
be very happy if publication of their major discoveries could appear at a scientific
meeting within a month of their presentation. Table 2.3 presents the chronological spread of the news of the discovery of the cause of tuberculosis.

The famous postulates of causation included in that paper consisted of only
one eight-line paragraph of that 17-page paper, and certainly did not appear to be
a major highlight at the time of presentation. As indicated earlier in this chapter,
most of the four criteria presented by Koch had been foreshadowed by Henle in
1840 and by Klebs in 1877, neither of whom was given credit in this paper. Koch
also did not mention Weigert, who had discovered the tissue-stain method he
employed, nor did he credit Tyndall for the culture medium he used to grow the
organism. However, Koch stated in regard to the method that "Its principle rests
on the use of a solid transport medium, which retains its solid consistency at
incubator temperature. The advantages of this method of pure culture which I
have introduced into bacteriology, I have explained in detail in an earlier publication" (Koch, 1932). Koch does refer to the fact that Klebs, Schuller, and Tous-
saint had previously cultivated microorganisms from tuberculous masses, but
Koch discards their findings as being on organisms other than the tubercle

Table 2.3
Chronology of Robert Koch's Discovery of the Cause of Tuberculosis[a]

August 18, 1881	Work began at Berlin Imperial Health Office
March 24, 1882	Presented proof that the tubercle bacillus caused tuberculosis at Berlin Physiological Society in Berlin
April 10, 1882	Work published in *Berliner Klinische Wochenschrift* **19:**221–230, 1882
April 20, 1882	Presented paper at First Congress of Internal Medicine, Weisbaden, April 20–22; Edwin Klebs present
April 22, 1882	Work translated by John Tyndall in England and published as letter in *London Times* with long editorial
May 3, 1882	Tyndall's letter republished by *New York Times*
May 3, 1882	*New York Tribune* publishes editorial suggesting application of Koch's findings to vaccine for TB

[a]Derived in part from Brock (1988), pp 117–132.

bacillus. His reason was that their organisms grew rapidly, producing early cloudiness of the medium, and were motile, whereas his organism grew very sparsely in liquids, never clouded it, was nonmotile, and became recognizable only after 3 or 4 weeks.

Earlier versions of the postulates had also appeared in Koch's work on anthrax in 1876 (Koch, 1876) and on wound infections in 1878 (Koch, 1878). The 1878 version as translated by Carter (1982) included the following three points: "1) The microorganism must be exhibited in all cases of the disease. 2) The distribution of the microorganism must correlate with and explain the course of the disease and the disease symptoms. 3) For each different disease, a morphologically distinguishable microorganism must be identified."

The 1882 version was as follows: "To prove that tuberculosis is a parasitic disease, that it is caused by the invasion of bacilli and that it is conditioned primarily by the growth and multiplication of the bacilli, it was necessary to isolate them from any disease-product of the animal organism which might adhere to them; and, by administering the isolated bacilli to animals, to reproduce the same morbid condition which, as known, is obtained by inoculation with spontaneously developed tuberculous material" (Koch, 1932).

The evidence that Koch presented to substantiate meeting the criteria in the postulates is summarized in Table 2.4 (see also Figure 2.4). As shown in the table, the presence of the organism in the lesions of the disease was established for both human and animal tuberculosis. The organism could be demonstrated in tissues from 30 out of 33 cases of human tuberculosis of various types. The three negatives were from cases of scrofulous lymph nodes or fungoid arthritis, of which Koch commented that the number examined was not large enough to determine whether they belong to true tuberculosis or not, although he felt that most of them probably did. In 34 cases of suspected tuberculosis in animals (including cows, monkeys, guinea pigs, rabbits, one chicken, and one hog), all were positive for the organism (Figure 2.5). The reproduction of tuberculosis in experimental animals was thereafter successfully achieved in all 172 guinea pigs, 32 rabbits, and 5 cats, using a wide variety of materials, including sputum, from humans, monkeys, rabbits, cattle, and guinea pigs. The results of 13 experiments reproducing the disease with pure cultures from a variety of human and animal sources and with various numbers of culture transfers and periods of growth in culture are summarized in Table 2.4. They involve different animal species, different routes of inoculation, and different amounts of inoculum. Control animals were inoculated with the same materials devoid of the culture fluid, albeit the number of controls was rather meager. All of the 62 animals inoculated with various materials by different routes eventually developed lesions in which presence of the organism could be demonstrated. Questionable or negative results were obtained in a number of white rats fed repeatedly over 2 months with substances containing the organism; five of the rats were then inoculated intra-

Table 2.4
Koch's Evidence that the Tubercle Bacillus Causes Tuberculosis; Presence of Organism and Reproduction in Experimental Animals

	Presence of organism in lesion	
	Number tested	**Number positive**
Human diseases		
Miliary tuberculosis	11	11
Bronchitis and pneumonia	12	12
Solitary lesion of brain	1	1
Intestinal tuberculosis	2	2
Scrofulous lymph nodes	3	2
Fungoid arthritis	4	2
	33	30
Animal diseases		
Perlsucht (TB) in cattle	10	10
Lungs of cattle	3	3
Lymph node from hog	1	1
Chicken with tuberculosis	1	1
Monkeys with tuberculosis	3	3
Guinea pigs with tuberculosis	9	9
Rabbits with tuberculosis	7	7
	34	34

	Reproduction of disease with tuberculous materials	
Animals inoculated	**Number tested**	**Number positive**
Guinea pigs	172	172
Rabbits	32	32
Cats	5	5
	209	209

		Reproduction of disease with pure cultures of organism				
		Inoculated group			**Control group**	
Experimental animal	**Number tested**	**Material**	**Days cultured**	**Number positive**	**Number tested**	**Number positive**
		Abdominal inoculations				
Guinea pigs	4	Human TB lungs	54	4	2	0
Guinea pigs	6	Ape with TB	95	6	2	0

(*continued*)

Table 2.4
(Continued)

| | Reproduction of disease with pure cultures of organism | | | | | |
| | Inoculated group | | | | Control group | |
Experimental animal	Number tested	Material	Days cultured	Number positive	Number tested	Number positive
Guinea pigs	5	Lung from cattle	72	5	1	0
Mice	4	Lung from monkey	113	4		
Hamster	1	Same as above		1		
		Anterior eye chamber inoculations				
Rabbits	3	Human lung	89	3		
Rabbits	2	Serum + culture	91	2	1	0
Rabbit	1	Needle prick pure serum + culture	18		1	0
Rabbits	6	Needle prick serum + culture	105	6		
Guinea pigs	10	Monkey TB	142	10	2	0
Rats	Many	Fed over 2 months with infected animals		±		
Rats	Many	Simple inoculation		0		
Rats	5	5 previously fed rats inoculated IP with culture derived from monkey TB		5		
Rabbits	4	Ear vein inoculation from monkey TB lung	178	4	2	0
Rabbits	3	Ear vein inoculation from human TB lung	103	3		

(continued)

Table 2.4
(Continued)

| | Reproduction of disease with pure cultures of organism | | | | | |
| | Inoculated group | | | | Control group | |
Experimental animal	Number tested	Material	Days cultured	Number positive	Number tested	Number positive
Rabbits	2	Control			2	0
Rabbits	3	Ear vein inoculation from Perlsucht (TB) lung from cattle	121	3		
Cats	2	Abdominal injection from monkey TB	163	2		
Bitch	1	Abdominal inoculation from human miliary TB	94	1		
Total	62̄			62*	11	0

*This excludes the white rats that were resistant when fed TB materials as well as on simple inoculation, but five of the fed rats developed TB after IP inoculation with cultured material. This table was derived from Koch (1882a).

peritoneally and subsequently developed tuberculosis. In one rabbit in which a very small amount of inoculum was inoculated into the anterior chamber, the development of tuberculosis was slow and the lesions were only local. Of the 11 control animals that were either uninoculated or received blood serum without the organism, all remained healthy and/or displayed no evidence of tuberculosis in their tissues.

   In his discussion, Koch excludes the possibility that the findings were the result of spontaneous tuberculosis or of chance, undesigned infection because (1) neither of these produce such massive eruption of tubercles in such a short time; (2) "control animals, which were treated in exactly the same way as the infected animals with only the single difference that they received no bacillary culture, remained healthy"; and (3) "in the case of numerous guinea pigs and rabbits, infected and injected with other substances in the same way, for other purposes of research, there never occurred this typical picture of miliary tuberculosis, which can only exist when the body is suddenly overwhelmed with a large number of bacilli."

As to the significance of the findings, Koch states: "If we ask further what significance belongs to the results gained in this study of tuberculosis, it must be considered a gain for science that it has been possible for the first time to establish the complete proof of the parasitic nature of a human infection, and this of the most important one. So far such proof was established only for anthrax, while in a number of other infectious diseases in human beings, for example, relapsing fever, wound infections, leprosy, gonorrhea, it was only known that parasites occur simultaneously with the pathological process, but the causal connection between the two has not been established" (Koch, 1932). He also expected that the study of tuberculosis would provide new viewpoints for other

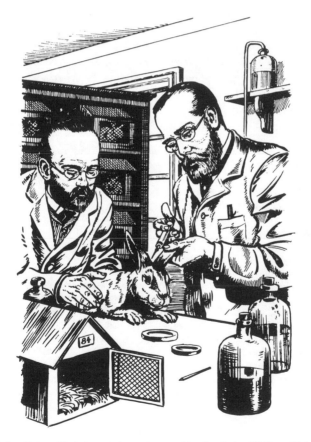

Figure 2.5.   Robert Koch inoculating animals with tubercle bacilli (from Knight, 1961).

infectious diseases and that the research methods used in tuberculosis would be of advantage in the investigation of other infectious diseases.

Finally, the importance of the findings in the control and prevention of tuberculosis was not lost upon Koch. He pointed out that knowledge of the tangible parasite causing tuberculosis will provide a favorable outlook for success in fighting the disease, first by controlling the source of infection, particularly the sputum; second, by disinfecting contaminated clothes, beds, etc.; and third, by controlling tuberculosis in animals. [Koch regarded meat and milk from animals infected with tuberculosis (Perlsucht) to be an important public health problem in the future.] These represent the substance of Koch's first report on tuberculosis.

In a second paper on tuberculosis presented by Koch in April 1882 (a month after the publication of his first paper) before physicians attending the first congress on internal medicine in Wiesbaden (Koch, 1882b), he explicitly stated his indebtedness to Klebs. Koch mentioned various methods used to prove causality and observed that "the best method, the method used by everyone who has been seriously occupied with these investigations was introduced and refined by Klebs." He then described the method by stating the criteria we know today as the postulates (Carter, 1982).

Klebs was present at that meeting, and a full translation* of his discussion of Koch's paper is quoted here because of its importance in establishing the priority of Kleb's earlier work.

> All of you will know that I have been involved with these issues since the 1860's. When I look back on all the hard labor that was involved over those years, with findings that are relatively unknown in medical circles, I am extremely pleased to welcome a method which allows us, in a much easier way, to establish the fact that tuberculosis is a disease caused by an infectious agent and to draw the proper conclusions from that insight.
>
> When I started my work in the field of tuberculosis, we were familiar with Villemin's attempts. His findings were not unambiguous, since the close relationship between the site of inoculation and the tuberculosis that resulted was not adequately stressed. In the past, I attempted to do so by following the development of tuberculosis, starting in the abdomen and continuing through lymphatic vessels of the diaphragm. In those earlier studies I could establish the basic patterns that Cohnheim later confirmed in more detail. My work was partly based on post-mortem findings. He has acknowledged that his views on this matter are basically similar to mine. But there is more. Following the scientific principles that have recently been developed by Koch, principles concerning the nature of an organism related to disease causation, I have tried to provide evidence that the poison that is the cause of tuberculosis can sustain and multiply outside the body.

---

*I am indebted to Dr. L. Lumey and to Dr. Mervin Susser, Columbia University School of Public Health, for providing this translation.

I have reported on my first successful attempts to inoculate this substance at the scientific meeting in Munich. I had prepared a follow-up article just before Koch's work was published. As always, I used egg yolk as the culture medium. In this medium centers of growth developed which were of different appearance than those described by Koch. And according to my analysis, they seemed to consist of micrococci. With these I have been able to bring about tuberculosis.

I do admit that the researches of Koch are in many aspects superior but I wish to make the claim that I was the first one who tried to grow these organisms outside the body, and that I was the first one to prove that these organisms, that can grow independently, are the carriers of the disease. This claim may be of minor importance but it *is* of personal importance to me. I mention this as an individual who is compelled to fight attacks from many sides. I do not wish to slight and devalue the work of Koch. Everyone who is involved in this field of research and all those who will benefit from this work owe a lot of gratitude to Koch. And I would like to thank Dr. Koch that he has kindly acknowledged my work in this field.

This gracious discussion of priority by Klebs could well be emulated by many competitive scientists today anxious to establish their claim to being first to identify the cause of a disease or a new methodology. It also emphasizes the fact that very few discoveries are made by investigators *de novo;* most build on the work or ideas of others who preceded them.

Table 2.2 presents a comparison of the contributions made by Klebs and by Koch.

The proof that the organism actually caused the disease was best stated in Koch's paper "Bacteriological Research," which he delivered at the 10th Internal Medical Congress in Berlin (Koch, 1892). Even there, it was not given major emphasis in his presentation and was only a small part of his discussion. The following is an excerpt from the original text in German:

Wenn es sich num aber nachweisen liess: erstens, dass der Parasit in jedem einzelnen Falle der betreffenden Krankheit anzutreffen ist, und zwar unter Verhaltnissen, welcheden pathlogiscehn Veranderungen und dem klinischen Verlauf der Krankheit entsprechen: zweitens, dass er bei keiner anderen Krankheit als zufalliger und nicht pathogener Schmarotzer vorkommt; und drittens, dass er, von dem Korper vollkommen isolirt und in Reinculturen hinreichend oft umgezuchtet, im Stande ist, von Neuem die Krankheit zu erzeugen; dann konnte er nicht mehr zufalliges Accidens der Krankheit sein, sondern liess sich in diesem Falle kein Anderes Verhaltnis mehr zwischen Parasit und Krankheit denken, als dass der Parasit die Ursache der Krankheit ist.

Translated into English, the three basic concepts are summarized in Table 2.5. Koch concluded that if all of the conditions could be satisfied, then the "occurrence of the parasite in the disease can no longer be accidental, but in this case no other relation between it and the disease except that the parasite is the cause of the disease can be considered." At the time of presentation, Koch felt that certain human and animal agents fully fulfilled these criteria. These included

Table 2.5
Henle–Koch Postulates[a]

---

1. The parasite occurs in every case of the disease in question and under circumstances which can account for the pathological changes and clinical course of the disease.
2. It occurs in no other disease as a fortuitous and nonpathogenic parasite.
3. After being fully isolated from the body and repeatedly grown in pure culture, it can induce the disease anew.

---

[a]Based on River's (1937) translation.

the organisms causing anthrax, tuberculosis, erysipelas, tetanus, and many animal diseases; in particular, almost all diseases that are infectious for animals.

At the same time, there were a number of infectious agents that did not meet all of the criteria, and that Koch felt were still strongly implicated in the causation of the disease. These included the bacteria isolated from typhoid fever, diphtheria, leprosy, relapsing fever, and Asiatic cholera. The major problem of fulfillment was the inability "to produce the disease anew" in an experimental host. Koch felt keenly that cholera was due to the vibrio because he himself had first discovered the organism (although the credit probably belongs to Pacini in 1854) and identified its constant relationship with the disease in an epidemic that he studied in Egypt and India (Koch, 1884). Yet there was no experimental animal in which the disease could be reproduced. As a matter of fact, Koch's contemporary, the great hygienist and chemist, Professor Max Pettenkofer of Munich, felt that the disease was not directly reproduced by the organism found in the stool, but required the acquisition of some factor of virulence through residence in the soil (the so-called Bodentheorie) (Pettenkofer, 1884, 1855; Howard-Jones, 1973). To prove this, Pettenkofer carried out his *experimentum crucium* in 1880. He swallowed 1.0 ml of a freshly grown broth culture from a case of cholera but did not develop the disease (Evans, 1973), even though he excreted large amounts of cholera vibrio, had gas and colic, and suffered from diarrhea for about a week. Despite showing these symptoms, he felt that his experiment established his view that cholera was not produced by the organism alone. Some of Pettenkofer's students did not fare quite as well and developed more severe illness when they later repeated the master's experiment. Pettenkofer did believe that the organism caused the disease, but only after it acquired virulence in the soil and in the presence of certain host factors. Despite John Snow's (1936) brilliant epidemiological proof of transmission by drinking water, Pettenkofer could neither reproduce these epidemiological observations in his studies of cholera epidemics in Germany, nor accept them on their own merits (Pettenkofer, 1884).

Another problem limiting the application of the Henle–Koch postulates was the inability to grow in the laboratory many presumed human pathogens, such as malaria and leprosy.

Thus, even at the time presented, the Henle–Koch postulates were never recommended as rigid criteria of causation. They failed to apply to many diseases at a time when a causal relationship with the organism isolated from them seemed almost unequivocal. Koch himself felt that fulfillment of the first two postulates might be sufficient evidence of causality.

The second criterion, that the organism "occurs in no other disease as a fortuitous and nonpathogenic parasite," became difficult to fulfill after it was found that an organism could also occur during or following asymptomatic infections, and sometimes persisted for months and even years. For example, during the prolonged asymptomatic or chronic carrier states of organism "A," a disease due to organism "B" might intervene, thus making organism "A" a fortuitous and nonpathogenic one in the presence of an unrelated disease. While suggested by Pettenkofer as early as 1855, the actual existence of such carriers was not acknowledged until 1893, when these carriers were recognized by Koch himself in his studies on cholera (Koch, 1893). The importance of carriers in the transmission of infection became abundantly clear with the work of Park and Beebe (1894) on diphtheria, of Koch (1903) on typhoid fever, and of Chapin (1910) on the control of communicable diseases.

Even today, almost 100 years after Koch's postulates were published, many bacterial causes of disease cannot fulfill his criteria despite enormous technical advances. Leprosy, syphilis, and malaria still elude growth in pure culture. Typhoid fever and leprosy cannot be reproduced in experimental animals with features resembling the human illness; neither can the newer organisms such as *Mycoplasma pneumoniae,* which causes an atypical pneumonia, or *Chlamydia trachomatis,* which is the major cause of nongonococcal urethritis and of bacterial pneumonia in infants. Further, while Koch felt that each infectious disease had a single cause, he did not recognize that one cause could produce several clinical syndromes (Evans, 1967). Other limitations of the Henle–Koch postulates for bacterial diseases will be discussed in Chapter 7.

New Diseases

While the details of the methodology will be discussed in more detail later in this book, examples will be presented here to illustrate the modern approach to establishing causation in bacterial diseases. The steps usually involve:

1. an epidemiological investigation to establish the source and method of transmission of the infecting agent
2. a laboratory investigation, often requiring exhaustive exploration of the

usefulness of older techniques and/or the development of new ones to isolate and grow the suspected causative agent from the presumed source of infection, from infected materials from the host, and/or isolation from the presumed vehicle of transmission

3. attempts to reproduce the disease with the cultured organisms in experimental animals, or, failing that and ethical considerations permitting, the reproduction in human volunteers

4. the use of case–control epidemiological techniques to demonstrate that the organism is present more often in cases than in controls, and the use of prospective studies to show that persons infected with the organism develop the disease, while those not infected do not (unless some other organism can result in the same clinical picture)

Two examples of new diseases are Legionnaire's disease (legionellosis) and Lyme disease.

Legionnaire's Disease

The annual convention of the Pennsylvania Department of the American Legion was held in Philadelphia from July 21 to July 24, 1976, with headquarters at the Bellevue-Stratford Hotel. Over the next four weeks, 221 persons who either had attended the convention or had been in or near the hotel developed pneumonia or other febrile diseases, and 34 died (Fraser *et al.*, 1977; Fraser, 1991). The disease was dubbed "Legionnaire's" pneumonia or disease.

Intensive epidemiological and laboratory investigations were initiated by the local and state health departments and by a team from the Centers for Disease Control (CDC) under the leadership of Dr. David Fraser (Figure 2.6). Because the initial attempts to isolate a causative agent failed, it was necessary to adopt an epidemiological definition based on the population at risk (the Legionnaires and their families), the time of exposure at the convention, and the clinical features of the disease. Using this as a guideline, a case–control comparison was made to identify the epidemiological characteristics of those with and without the disease. It was found that delegates to the convention who resided in the Bellevue-Stratford Hotel and older males who smoked were at highest risk for the disease. Since no evidence of person-to-person transmission could be identified and a common source in food could be excluded, an airborne source was suspected. This was supported by the increased risk among those who spent time in the lobby of the Bellevue-Stratford Hotel. Such a source seemed even more likely when it was found that the disease was occurring among non-Legionnaires who had simply walked past the hotel on Broad Street or had watched a parade from there.

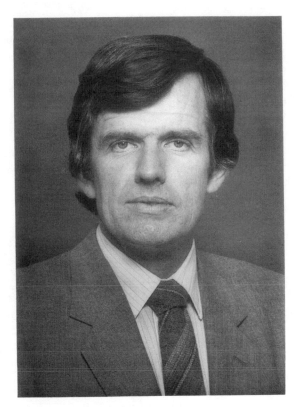

Figure 2.6. Dr. David W. Fraser, 1944– , Head, Social Welfare Department, Secretariat of His Royal Highness the Aga Khan, Paris, France.

After 5 months of intensive laboratory investigation, McDade and associates (1979) at CDC finally identified a fastidious gram-negative rod in inoculated guinea pigs, using techniques similar to those commonly employed for rickettsial studies. The organism was named *Legionella pneumophilia*. Successful bacterial media were then developed for its growth, and an immunofluorescent serological test for diagnosis and survey work was established. Direct identification of the organism by immunofluorescence in the lung at autopsy, the isolation of the organism from respiratory secretions, lung tissue, and the blood of patients with Legionnaire's pneumonia, and the much higher prevalence of antibody in cases than in controls helped to establish the causal relationship. The disease could eventually be reproduced in guinea pigs, with cultured materials. The Koch postulates were therefore fulfilled. Many strains of the organism have now been identified. One causes a pneumonia called Pittsburgh pneumonia and another causes explosive outbreaks of a febrile disease without pneumonia, termed Pontiac fever. Prior outbreaks in 1965 in a Washington hospital (Thacker *et al.*, 1978), in the same Philadelphia hotel in 1974 (Terranova *et al.*, 1978), and in a meat-packing plant way back in 1957 (Osterholm, 1983) have been identified, using stored serum samples. The organism exists in the soil and contaminates cooling water towers from where it is disseminated by air-conditioning equipment in hotels, hospitals, and other institutions, as well perhaps by contaminated shower heads. While a cell membrane fraction containing lipid, carbohydrate, and protein derived from the organism has been shown to induce the production of antibodies in experimental animals and to protect them against subsequent infections with the same living organisms, the introduction of such a cell membrane fraction has not been attempted in humans.

Lyme Disease

In October 1945, two mothers from Lyme, Connecticut, a small coastal community of 5000 people, reported to the State Health Department that 12 children in their community who lived close together had an illness diagnosed as juvenile rheumatoid arthritis (JRA). To investigate this, a surveillance system was set up by the Health Department and the Yale University Rheumatology Section through contacts with mothers, area physicians, school nurses, and local health officials in the three contiguous communities of Old Lyme, Lyme, and East Kaddam (total population 12,000). All cases with inflammatory joint disease were sought and invited to come to the Yale Clinic for evaluation and study. The first reports in 1976 and 1977 by Steere (Figure 2.7) and coworkers included 39 children and 12 adults who had a similar type of arthritis, with brief but recurrent attacks of asymmetric swelling and pain in the large joints over a period of years. The key clinical finding was that an erythematous papule, consistent with an insect bite, that developed into an expanding, red annular lesion had occurred in 13 (25%) of the patients during a median period of 4 weeks before the onset of arthritis; only 2 of the 159 family members of patients had such a lesion but did *not* develop arthritis ($p < 0.0000001$). Only one patient remembered being bitten by a tick. The skin lesion most closely resembled erythema chronicum migrans disease (ECM or EMD), described in Europe in 1909 and known to be associated with a tick bite and with subsequent neurological abnormalities, but not with arthritis.

Epidemiological studies on Lyme arthritis in 12 contiguous Connecticut communities revealed geographic and familial clustering, a seasonal occurrence mostly between May 1 and November 30, and an age range from 2 to 83 years (median age 28 years), with about equal sex distribution. A case–control study of ECM and Lyme arthritis was carried out among 43 residents and 64 neighborhood controls in the fall of 1977 (Steere *et al.*, 1978). The major findings of

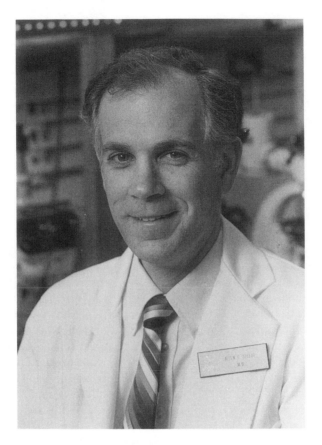

Figure 2.7. Dr. Allen Steere, 1943– , Professor of Medicine, Tufts University School of Medicine.

statistical significance between cases and controls were the presence of cats in the homes of more patients than controls (63% versus 39%), the presence of ticks on pets (70% for patients versus 27% for controls), a history of tick bites in 1977 (44% versus 26%), and the presence of farm animals (26% versus 11%). The incidence of the disease in 1977 was 2.8 cases per 1000 residents in three communities on the east side of the Connecticut River, while it was 0.1 case per 1000 residents in the nine communities on the west side, a difference of almost 30-fold. These initial clinical and epidemiological findings pointed to the cause as an infectious, tick-borne agent, most probably a virus. Extensive isolation and serological studies for a wide variety of microbial causes were carried out and were all negative, including tests for 216 arboviruses, 38 of which were known to be tick transmitted. When it was found that patients with Lyme arthritis responded to penicillin or tetracycline therapy, as suggested by results in Europe with ECM, a viral etiology was excluded (Steere *et al.*, 1983). In further case studies, the clinical spectrum was extended to neurological and cardiac manifestations, and the designation was changed to Lyme disease to reflect this multisystem involvement (Reik *et al.*, 1979; Steere *et al.*, 1980).

A cohort study of 314 patients in Connecticut from 1976 through 1982 confirmed the previous studies and outlined the early clinical manifestations (Steere *et al.*, 1983). Meanwhile, Burgdorfer and his associates at the Rocky Mountain Laboratories in Montana were pursuing the possible spirochetal causation of ECM, based on suggestions made as early as 1948 (Lennhoff 1948; Hollstrom, 1930, 1958). Using *Ixales dammini* ticks from Shelter Island, New York, where Lyme disease was known to be endemic, Burgdorfer *et al.* (1982) identified spirochetelike organisms by staining the dissected organs with Giemsa or by darkfield examination. Of 124 ticks, 75 (60%) were found to contain the organism, mostly in the midgut. In addition to this, sera from 9 patients were found, through immunofluorescence, to contain antibody (Burgdorfer *et al.*, 1982).

Based on these findings, Steere and his group were able to isolate the organism from the blood, skin lesions, or cerebral fluid of 3 out of 56 patients (5.4%), using a modified Kelly's medium, and were able to demonstrate antibody increases against the agent. The antibody changes included the demonstration of IgM-type antibody in 36 out of 40 cases with early ECM illness, as compared with 3 out of 20 control patients with infectious mononucleosis. IgG antibody was found in 89 out of 95 cases (93.7%) with later manifestations of the disease, as compared with 0 out of 80 control patients. In the same issue of the *New England Journal of Medicine,* Benach *et al.* (1983) reported the isolation of the organism from the blood of two other patients. Steere *et al.* summarized their isolation attempts in the first international symposium on the disease. Only 4 isolates had been obtained from 118 patients on whom cultures were done and none were from the synovium or synovial fluid involved in the arthritic manifestations, even though immune complexes have been demonstrated. An international symposium on Lyme disease has now been held and the proceedings published (Steere, 1984).

While the spirochetal causation (or more properly, borrelia causation) of ECM and Lyme disease is widely accepted, the current evidence does not fulfill Koch's postulates. The parasite is not demonstrable in every case of the disease, being found in less than 3% of the cases thus far tested. This may be because the isolation technique is not sensitive enough, or the organism has disappeared by the time the sample is obtained. The failure to isolate the organism from the joints and failure to show a persistent spirochetemia makes it difficult to prove that the parasite "can account for the pathological changes and the clinical course of the disease," as required by the postulates. The immunopathological nature of the pathogenesis of the disease may explain both of these missing factors. The organism has now been grown in pure culture, including solid media, but the disease has not been fully reproduced in an experimental animal with such a culture. Rabbits can be infected and develop a rash but they do not develop the later manifestations. An earlier study did report the transmission of ECM to volunteers by transfer of biopsies of lesions from patients (Binder *et al.*, 1955), but the possible spirochetal etiology was unknown at the time. The antibody evidence on which much of the causal proof rested was, of course, based on knowledge unknown to Koch at the time of his postulates. While antibody to *Borrelia burgdorferi* of both the IgG and IgM types appears frequently during illness, there is much irregularity in its demonstration. A highly sensitive, standardized, and repeatable laboratory test is also lacking. Osterholm *et al.* (1991) found that only 10 out of 29 cases of Lyme disease with the typical rash, erythema chronica migracans, had either an elevated acute or convalescent antibody titer; other studies quoted by him have reported an elevated IgM titer in only 8 out of 22 patients during acute illness, although ultimately, all showed at least one elevated IgM or IgG titer at some point in the illness. Final proof will rest on prospective epidemiological studies showing that only persons who develop the infection lack specific antibody (using a reliable test), develop it regularly during illness, and are then protected against reinfection by the presence of such antibody. Persons lacking antibody to the agent should be susceptible to the disease. An animal model for Lyme arthritis has now been developed (Barthold *et al.*, 1988) that is being used to test the efficiency of an experimental vaccine. Encouraging steps toward the development of a human vaccine and the use of the polymerase chain reaction to identify the antigen in affected tissues may also soon further strengthen the causal relationship.

References

Barthold SW, Moody KP, Twillinger CA, *et al:* An animal model for Lyme arthritis. *Ann NY Acad Sci* **539:**264–273, 1988.

Baumgartner I: Edwin Klebs: A centennial note. *N Engl J Med* **213:**60–63, 1935.

Benach J, Bosler E, Hanrahan J, *et al:* Spirochetes isolated from the blood of two cases with Lyme disease. *N Engl J Med* **309:**740–742, 1983.

Binder E, Doepfer R and Hornstein O: Experimentalle ubertragund des erythema chronicum migrans von mench zu mench. *Hautzart* **6:**494–496, 1955.

Brock TD: *Robert Koch: A Life in Medicine and Bacteriology.* Madison, Wisconsin, Science Tech Publishing, 1988.

Bulloch W: *The History of Bacteriology.* London, Oxford University Press, 1938.

Burgdorfer W, Barbour A, Hayes SF, *et al:* Lyme disease—A tick borne spirochetosis? *Science* **216:**1317–1319, 1982.

Carter KC: Klebs and Koch's postulates. *ASM News* **49:**142, 1982.

Castiglione A: *A History of Medicine.* New York, Knopf, 1947.

Chapin CV: *The Sources and Modes of Transmission of Infection.* New York, Wiley and Co, 1910.

Craft JE, Grodzicki RL, Steere AC: Antibody response in Lyme disease. Evaluation of diagnostic tests. *J Infect Dis* **149**:789–795, 1984.

Doetsch RN: Koch's postulates. *ASM News* **48**:555–556, 1982.

Evans AS: Clinical syndromes in adults caused by respiratory infection. *Med Clin N Amer* **51**:803–815, 1967.

Evans AS: Pettenkofer revisited. The life and contributions of Max von Pettenkofer (1818–1901). *Yale J Biol Med* **46**:161–176, 1973.

Evans AS: Causation and disease. The Henle–Koch postulates revisited. *Yale J Biol Med* **49**:175–195, 1976.

Foster WD: *A History of Bacteriology and Immunology.* London, Wm Heinemann Medical Books, 1970.

Fraser D: Legionellosis, in Evans AS, Brachman PA (eds): *Bacterial Infections of Humans: Epidemiology and Control,* 2nd ed. New York, Plenum Press, 1991, pp 333–347.

Fraser DW, Tsai TR, Orenstein W, *et al:* Legionnaire's disease—Description of an epidemic of pneumonia. *N Engl J Med* **297**:1189–1197, 1977.

Henle J: *Pathologische Untesuchen.* Berlin: A Hirschwold, 1840, pp 1–82.

Henle J: *On Miasmata and Contagie,* Rosen G (trans). Baltimore, Johns Hopkins University Press, 1938.

Hollstrom E: Erythema chronica migrans Afzeli. *Acta Derm Venereol* **11**:315–321, 1930.

Hollstrom E: Penicillin treatment of erythema chronicum migrans Afzelius. *Acta Derm Venereol* **38**:285–289, 1958.

Howard-Jones N: Gelsenkirchen typhoid epidemic of 1901, Robert Koch, and the dead hand of Max von Pettenkofer. *Br Med J* **1**:103, 1973.

Howard-Jones N: Fracastoro and Henle: A reappraisal of their contributions to the concept of communicable diseases. *Med Hist* **21**:61–68, 1977.

Klebs E: Uber Tuberkulose. Munich, *Amtl Bericht ver Versamulung, Deutsch Naturforsch Aerzte* **50**:274, 1877.

Klebs E: Die Blindschleichen Tuberkelbazillen und ihre Verwendung bei menschlichen und Warmbluter-Tuberkulose. Berlin, Deutsche Aerzte-zig, 1908, p 457.

Knight D: *Robert Koch, Father of Bacteriology.* New York, F. Watts, 1961.

Koch R: Verfrahren zur Untersuchung zur conserviren und photographie der Bakterien, Beitrag der Pflanzen. Cohn's Bier. 2 Morph Pflanzen, Breslow 1876, vol 2, pp 399–434.

Koch R: Untersuchen uber die Aetiologie der Wundinfectionokrankheiten, in Cheyne WW (trans): *Investigations into the Etiology of Traumatic Infective Diseases by R. Koch.* London: New Syndenham Society, 1880, vol 88, p 1.

Koch R: 1843–1903: The etiology of anthrax, 1877. The etiology of tuberculosis, 1882a. Baltimore, Williams & Wilkins, 1938.

Koch R: Uber die Atiologie der Tuberkulose. Verhandlungen des Kongresses fur inner Medicin. Erste Kongress. Wiesbaden, Verlag von JF Bergmann, 1882b, pp 56–66.

Koch R: Uber die Cholerabakterien. *Dtsch Med Wochenschr* **10**:725–728, 1884.

Koch R: Uber bakteriologische forschung, in: *Vehr X Int Cong.* Berlin, 1892, p 95.

Koch R: Uber den augenblichen stand in bacteriologische cholera-diagnose. *J Hyg Infectionskrankh* **14**:393–426, 1893.

Koch R: Die Bekampfung des Typhus. Veroffentlichungen auf dem Gebiete des Militarischen Sanitats-Wesens Vol 21 Hirchwald, Berlin Gessammelte Werke 2/1, 1903, pp 296–305.

Koch R: Die aetiologie der milzbrand krankheiten begrunded auf die entwicklungegeschichte des *Bacillus anthracis* 1876. Eingeleitet de M Fischer, JA Barth, 1910.

Koch R: *The Aetiology of Tuberculosis,* Dr and Mrs Max Pinner (trans). *Am Rev Tuber,* 1932.

Lennhoff C: Spirochete in aetiologically obscure diseases. *Acta Derm Venereol* **28**:295–324, 1948.

McDade JE, Shepard CC, Fraser DW, *et al:* Legionnaire's disease: Isolation of a bacterium and demonstration of its role in other respiratory disease. *N Engl J Med* **297**:1197–1203, 1977.

McDade JE, Brenner DJ, Bozeman FM: Legionnaire's disease bacterium isolated in 1947. *Ann Intern Med* **90**:659–661, 1979.

Osterholm MT, Chin TD, Osborne DO, *et al:* A 1957 outbreak of Legionnaire's disease associated with a meat packing plant. *Am J Epidemiol* **117**:60–67, 1983.

Osterholm MT, MacDonald KL, Hedberg CW: Lyme disease, in Evans AS, Brachman PA (eds): *Bacterial Infections of Humans: Epidemiology and Control,* 2nd ed. New York, Plenum Press, 1991, pp 403–423.

Park W, Beebe AL: Diphtheria and pseudodiphtheria. *Med Rec* **46**:385–481, 1894.

Pettenkofer M: Cholera. *Lancet* **2**:769–776, 816–819, 904–905, 992–994, 1042–1043, 1086–1088, 1884.

Pettenkofer M: *Untersuchen und Becbachtungen uber die Verbreitsungs art Einhalt zu thun uber Massregeln derselben.* TG Cottascher, Buchhandlung, Munich, 1885.

Reik L, Steere AD, Bartenhazen NH, *et al:* Neurological manifestations of Lyme disease. *Medicine* **58**:281–294, 1979.

Rivers T: Virus and Koch's postulates. *J Bacteriol* **33**:1–12, 1979.

Snow J: *On the Communication of Cholera.* London, Churchill, 1849.

Snow J: *On the Communication of Cholera* 2nd ed. London, Churchill, 1855.

Snow J: On the mode of communication of cholera, in: *Snow on cholera.* New York, The Commonwealth Fund, 1936, pp 1–175.

Steere AC, Maliwista SE, Syndman DR: A cluster of arthritis in children and adults in Lyme, Connecticut (abstract). *Arthritis Rheum* **19**:824, 1976.

Steere A, Maliwista S, Syndman D, *et al:* Lyme arthritis. An epidemic of oliogoarticular arthritis in children and young adults in three Connecticut communities. *Arthritis Rheum* **20**:7–17, 1977.

Steere A, Broderick T, Maliwista S: Erythema chronicum migrans and Lyme arthritis. Epidemiologic evidence for a tick vector. *Am J Epidemiol* **108**:312–321, 1978.

Steere A, Taylor E, Wilson M, *et al:* Longitudinal assessment of the clinical and epidemiological features of Lyme disease in a community. *J Infect Dis* **154**:295–300, 1980.

Steere AC, Maliswista SE, Croft JE, *et al* (eds): First International Symposium on Lyme Disease. *Yale J Biol Med* **57**:445–714, 1982.

Steere AC, Grodzicki MS, Kornblatt AN, *et al:* The spirochetal etiology of Lyme disease. *N Engl J Med* **308**:733–740, 1983.

Terranova W, Cohen ML, Fraser DW: 1974 outbreak of Legionnaires' disease 1977: Clinical and epidemiological features. *Lancet* **2**:122–124, 1978.

Thacker SB, Bennett JV, Tsai TF, *et al:* An outbreak in 1965 of severe respiratory disease caused by the Legionnaires' disease bacterium. *J Infect Dis* **138**:512–519, 1978.

Causation and Acute
Viral Diseases

The discovery of viruses, their growth in mice, in tissue culture, and in embryo-
nated eggs brought new problems in causation and reemphasized the limitations
of the original Henle–Koch postulates. Dr. Thomas Rivers (Figure 3.1), the
distinguished American virologist, discussed these issues in his presidential address before the American Society of Immunology in 1937 (Rivers, 1937). Dr.
Rivers had headed the virology research program at the Rockefeller Foundation
and, with Frank Horsfall, had edited one of the first great texts in virology
(Rivers and Horsfall, 1959). In his lecture, he pointed out that blind adherence to
Koch's postulates might sometimes act as a hindrance rather than an aid. For
example, the idea that an infectious malady can be caused only by the action of a
single agent is incorrect. If Shope had adhered to this notion, he would never
have discovered that swine influenza as it occurs in nature is caused by the
combined or synergistic action of two agents, one a virus not cultivable on
lifeless media, the other an ordinary hemophilic bacterium (Shope, 1931). The
requirement that the infectious agent be grown in a pure state on lifeless media
also hindered the establishment of the causal relation of viruses to disease,
because viruses require living tissues for propagation, as in chick embryo or
tissue culture. Thus, Rivers felt that "Koch's postulates have not been fulfilled in
viral diseases." In their place he suggested the conditions to be met before the
specific relation of a virus to a disease is established (Table 3.1). In these criteria
Rivers felt that it is not essential that a virus be grown on lifeless carriers or in
modified tissue cultures. In illness, the specific causative virus should always be
found at the proper time in specific lesions. In establishing proof of causation,
animals should become sick or die when inoculated with material from such
tissues shown to be free of ordinary microbes or rickettsiae and it should be
possible to transmit the disease serially. Rivers warned that one must be wary in
doing this experiment, as experimental animals are subject to their own viral
diseases, and as such a different agent might be picked up during passage. The

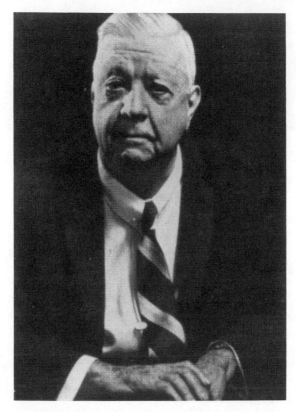

Figure 3.1. Thomas Milton Rivers, 1888–1962, Director of Virology, Rockefeller Institute of Medical Research (from Evans, 1976).

occurrence of healthy viral carrier states in experimental animals may also lead to picking up the wrong agent in passage. External infection with other viruses being worked on within the laboratory may also occur.

Rivers also emphasized that in addition to recognition and isolation of the virus, "information concerning the presence of antibodies against the agent and the time of their appearance in the serum of patients is equally important as evidence of etiological significance of the virus" (Rivers, 1937). He pointed out that "if a virus is the actual cause of a disease, immune substances are virtually absent from the patient's serum at the onset of illness and make their appearance during the period of recovery." He also recognized that recovery sometimes occurs without the development of antibodies, and occasionally a person possessing antibodies against a virus succumbs to a disease caused by it. These immunological aspects of causation suggested by Rivers are important to emphasize

Table 3.1
Rivers's Conditions for Establishing Specific Relation of a Virus to a Disease[a]

1. A specific virus must be found associated with a disease with a degree of regularity.
2. The virus must be shown to occur in the sick individual not as an incidental or accidental finding but as the cause of the disease under investigation.

[a]From Rivers (1937).

because of later problems in viral disease in which the agent could not be isolated or transmitted to laboratory animals, and where proof of causation rested solely on these immunological criteria.

The Epidemiological Concept

While the Henle–Koch postulates involved the bacterial agent in causation, and Rivers added elements of virological and immunological proof, it was Dr. Robert J. Huebner (Figure 3.2) who emphasized another ingredient, the need for epidemiological data, in establishing causation in viral diseases (Huebner, 1957). Dr. Huebner had worked at the National Institutes of Health on several infectious diseases, including key investigations of Q fever. He later went on to make fundamental contributions to our knowledge of the relationship of RNA viruses to cancer, and to propose the concept of an oncogene in normal cells. In a 1957 paper entitled "The Virologist's Dilemma" (Huebner, 1957), he discussed the criteria for etiological association of prevalent viruses with prevalent diseases. In his view, the mere isolation of a viral agent having a temporal relation to the disease process, while necessary and important, provided a very low order of evidence for the purpose of proving causality. The virologist's dilemma was that improved technology had reduced "the isolation of new human and animal viruses from a technological feat of high order to an almost exasperating commonplace occurrence." At least 50 new viruses of man had been discovered and new and untyped agents by the hundreds were accumulating in freezers in virus laboratories far more rapidly than they could be characterized, classified, or associated in a meaningful way with the causation of specific diseases. A number of viruses such as those in the Coxsackie, enteric cytopathogenic human orphan viruses (ECHO), and adenovirus groups not only cause illness but also occur commonly in apparently healthy persons, i.e., a viral flora. Indeed, in one nursery studied by Huebner, all 43 infants were completely healthy in September

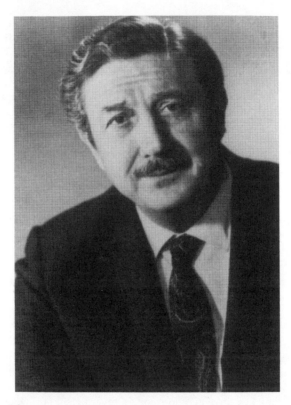

Figure 3.2. Robert J. Huebner, 1914– , former Chief, Laboratory of RNA Tumor Viruses, National Cancer Institute, National Institutes of Health (from Evans, 1976).

1955, yet all were carrying an ECHO-like virus, which was isolated on 90 occasions in that single month. In subsequent months, the nursery returned to a more "normal" state with high weekly rates of febrile illness.

This same high frequency of minor illnesses and a plethora of prevalent viruses have also been found in family settings in New Orleans, New York, and Seattle by Fox in a series of excellent studies carried out in these cities over several years under the heading "The Virus Watch Program" (Fox and Hall, 1980). These observations of wide dissemination, high prevalence, numerous immunological types, and frequent isolation of viruses from persons who were healthy or had only mild illnesses led Huebner to make a list of suggestions for establishing causality that incorporated elements of both Koch's and Rivers's postulates. He suggested these might be called a "Bill of Rights for Prevalent Viruses" to bring a legal concept to an area of scientific research and to comprise a guarantee against "the imputation of guilt by simple association." These conditions are outlined in Table 3.2, along with his comments. He also emphasized the need for specific hyperimmune sera against newly recognized viruses as a means of identifying and classifying them. Huebner cautioned that his suggestions should not be regarded as "postulates" or even as advice to forlorn virologists, but merely as useful guidelines.

As the causative agent of many specific clinical entities became established, it became apparent in 1960 that a number of common illnesses or syndromes existed in which several agents could produce the same clinical picture (Evans, 1967). It was also recognized that despite intensive investigation, no causative agent could be identified in 25–50% of common acute respiratory syndromes, in 75% or so of acute febrile clinical syndromes involving the central nervous

Table 3.2
Huebner's Prescription for the Virologist's Dilemma: Conditions Necessary for Establishing a Virus as Cause of a Specific Human Disease[a]

1. Virus must be a "real" entity: A new virus must be well established by passage in the laboratory in animal or tissue cultures.
2. Origin of virus: the virus must be repeatedly isolated from human specimens and shown not to be a viral contaminant of the experimental animals, cells, or media employed to grow it.
3. Antibody response: An increase in neutralizing or other serologically demonstrable antibodies should regularly result from active infection.
4. Characterization and comparison with known agents: A new virus should be fully characterized and compared with other agents including host and host-cell ranges, pathological lesions, types of cytopathogenic effects, size, susceptibility to physical agents, etc.
5. Constant association with specific illness: The virus must be constantly associated with any well-defined clinical entity and isolated from diseased tissue, if available.
6. Studies with human volunteers: Human beings inoculated with a newly recognized agent in "double-blind" studies should reproduce the clinical syndrome.
7. Epidemiological studies: Both "cross-sectional" and "longitudinal" studies of community or institutional groups to identify patterns of infection and disease.
8. Prevention by a specific vaccine: One of the best ways to establish an agent as the cause.
9. Financial support: A consideration so absolutely necessary that it deserves to be called a postulate.

[a]From Huebner (1957).

Table 3.3
The Five Realities of Acute Respiratory Disease[a]

1. The same clinical syndrome may be produced by a variety of agents.
2. The same etiological agent may produce a variety of clinical syndromes.
3. The predominating agent in a given clinical syndrome may vary according to the age group involved, the year, the geographic location, and the type of population (military or civilian).
4. Diagnosis of the etiological agent is frequently impossible on the basis of the clinical finding alone.
5. The cause (or causes) of a large percentage of common infectious disease syndromes is still unknown.

[a]From Evans (1967).

system, or in most cases of common acute gastroenteritis (now reduced to about 50% or less with the discovery of rota and Norwalk viruses). This led to my formulation of a group of "Five Realities" for acute respiratory disease, shown in Table 3.3 (Evans, 1967). These concepts greatly complicated establishing proof of causation; it became possible to state only that a given virus or other infectious agent was one of the causes of a given respiratory, gastrointestinal, or central nervous system syndrome, and that its causal involvement might be apparent only in certain years, or months of a year, or in certain age groups, or in military personnel and not in civilian populations, etc. For example, rhinoviruses are associated with only 20–25% of the common cold syndrome and are active mostly in the fall. Respiratory syncytial virus is the major cause of severe respiratory disease in infants, but it produces mild or even asymptomatic infections in older children and adults. Adenovirus types 4 and 7 are very important causes of acute respiratory disease in military recruits, but are of little consequence in young adults in civilian settings.

Thus, the establishment of a causal relationship of a given virus with a given syndrome became possible only under a set of special circumstances. The Henle–Koch postulates were concerned primarily with the nature of the agent in establishing causality; further than this, there was the need to consider the circumstances under which infection occurred; and finally, the influence of the host was recognized as important in determining whether clinical disease developed after infection occurred, since so many viral infections are asymptomatic.

Agents in Search of Disease

While the development and utilization of the chick embryo, suckling mice, and of tissue culture techniques for the isolation of viruses led to the discovery of a multitude of agents for which causal relationships to disease had to be worked out, technological developments in the late 1960s and early 1970s created a new problem. These new techniques permitted identification of a new agent by the electron microscope or by serological techniques, even though the agent itself could not be isolated and/or propagated in the laboratory. This made it impossible to apply Henle–Koch's, Rivers's, or Huebner's guidelines on causation. In some instances the "agent" identified was found in healthy persons or in persons with a chronic disease, and so the relationship to an acute infectious disease, if any, was not immediately apparent. The two best examples of this situation were first, the discovery of Australia antigen in 1964 by Blumberg (Figure 3.3) and his group (Blumberg *et al.*, 1964) in the serum of healthy aboriginal natives of Australia through immunodiffusion techniques, and second, the demonstration of herpeslike particles under the electron microscope by Epstein (Figure 3.4), Achong and Barr (1964) in cells cultured from a biopsy of an African lymphatic tumor described by Burkitt (1958). In neither instance could the "agent" be isolated or grown in pure culture in the laboratory.

The discovery of Australia antigen was made during genetic studies of disturbances in the proteins of human serum by Dr. Blumberg and his group at

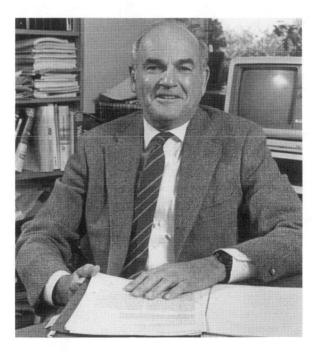

Figure 3.3. Dr. Baruch Blumberg, 1925– , Distinguished Scientist, Fox–Chase Cancer Center, Professor, University of Pennsylvania.

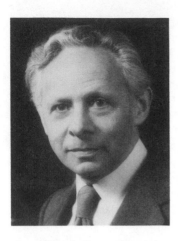

Figure 3.4. Sir Anthony Epstein, 1921–, Nuffield Department of Clinical Medicine, John Radcliffe Hospital, Oxford.

the University of Pennsylvania. In the course of analyzing sera from individuals of different ethnic groups, they encountered one serum from an Australian aborigine that was distinctly different from the lipoprotein precipitins previously found, and to which they gave the name "Australia antigen" (Blumberg *et al.*, 1964). The serological technique for identifying Australia antigen in the serum of human populations was simple enough to permit an epidemiological search for possible diseases to which it might be related. This approach is the opposite of the usual search for the causative agent of a given disease, since here we have an agent in search of the disease (if any) with which it is associated. A protocol for this type of study for specific antigen or antibody in population groups is outlined in Table 3.4. Tests for the prevalence of antigen in different population groups around the world were examined: the antigen was rare in population groups in the United States but had about 20% prevalence in sera from Peruvian Indians, although this provided no lead as to the associated disease.

Blumberg's group then tested sera from patients with a variety of infectious and chronic diseases. A high frequency of antigenemia was identified in persons with leukemia, Down's syndrome (mongolism), and viral hepatitis (Blumberg *et al.*, 1965, 1967). The final relationship to type B viral hepatitis was established by Prince (1968) and others (Okoche and Murakami, 1968). The relationship of the antigen to leukemia was observed in transfusions derived from antigen-positive donors, and that with Down's syndrome, in the close contact with a genetically susceptible population, in which antigenemia persisted. Further support for causation came from the longitudinal studies of Krugman and Giles at Willowbrook School and from their deliberate exposure experiments (Krugman *et al.*, 1967; Giles *et al.*, 1969). Subtypes of the antigen are now recognized, sensitive methods of detecting and screening for both hepatitis antigen and antibody have been developed (McCollum, 1982), and most important, an effective vaccine has been prepared, based on the original observations of Krugman (Figure 3.5) and his group at Willowbrook (Krugman *et al.*, 1970), and is now commercially available. The evidence for the relationship of Australia antigen, or hepatitis B virus (HBV), as it is now known, to hepatitis, rests on both virological and epidemiological data. The virological evidence consists of the almost constant presence of the antigen in the blood during the acute stages of the disease and the subsequent appearance of specific antibody. Epidemiological studies of the case–control, cross-sectional, and prospective types have established the association of the antigen and antibody to the disease. Most impressive is the demonstration that screening of blood donors to remove those that carry the antigen prevents the transfusion of hepatitis B and that a vaccine prepared from the blood of infected volunteers prevents the disease (Szmuness *et al.*, 1973). Molecular virological techniques inserting the HBV-DNA of the virus into yeast cells or vaccinia virus as a carrier particle of the antigen has proved to be effective, thus establishing the highly specific protection provided by the presumed causative agent. The proofs still needed to fulfill previous postulates of causation are the ability to grow the virus in the laboratory and to produce the *clinical* illness in an experimental animal (nonhuman primates such as the marmoset and the chimpanzee become infected after inoculation with serum from patients, as demonstrated by antigenemia and the development of antibody, but show no clinical symptoms). However, human volunteers inoculated with the

Table 3.4
Protocol for Seroepidemiological Pursuit of Agents in Search of Disease

1. Develop a serological technique that is simple, specific, and sensitive enough to be applied on a large scale to epidemiological investigation.
2. Determine the prevalence of the component in sera obtained from different geographic areas, age and sex groups, and socioeconomic settings to learn its distribution in healthy population groups.
3. Test acute and convalescent sera from different clinical syndromes, especially those of unknown cause in which there is some ground for suspecting a causal relationship.
4. If an association with a disease is found:
    A. Establish the specificity of the association and of the antibody produced.
    B. Initiate prospective studies.
        i. To show that persons possessing antibody are immune, those lacking it are susceptible;
        ii. To determine the incidence of infection and of disease in persons lacking antibody.

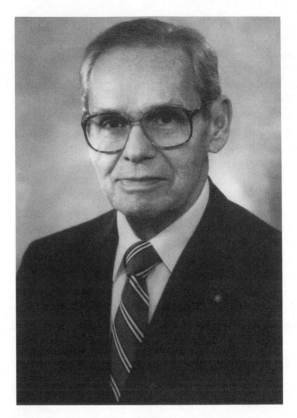

Figure 3.5. Dr. Saul Krugman, 1911– , Professor of Pediatrics, emeritus, New York University College of Medicine, New York.

antigen do become infected, and some of them develop the full clinical picture. For his discovery and work on Australia antigen and on viral hepatitis, Blumberg received the Nobel Prize in 1982. The strong relationship of hepatitis B virus to hepatocellular carcinoma will be discussed in a later chapter.

In 1968 the grandson of Jacob Henle, Dr. Werner Henle of Philadelphia (Figure 3.6), made a claim of causality that met none of the famous Henle–Koch postulates (Henle *et al.,* 1968). With his wife, Gertrude, and a young German physician, Volker Diehl, he claimed that Epstein–Barr virus (EBV), or a close relative of it, was the cause of infectious mononucleosis. The Henles had been born in Germany and came to this country to work in the virology laboratory of the Children's Hospital in Philadelphia. There, they did excellent studies on many viruses, including mumps, influenza, and viral hepatitis, before becoming involved with EBV. Their major technical development was an immunofluorescence test for EBV antibody (Henle and Henle, 1966). With this test, they carried out seroepidemiological studies in various groups. They found that the antibody was always present in African children with Burkitt's lymphoma, usually in very high titer, and was also present in some 80% of healthy African children. What was surprising was the common presence of the antibody in children and adults in the United States, suggestive of a common communicable disease of childhood. But what was the disease? Again, here we have an agent in search of a disease. Because the agent could not be isolated in tissue culture, the investigators had to rely on serological evidence.

The age pattern of antibody prevalence of EBV resembled that of other common viruses, such as those causing measles, mumps, and poliomyelitis in the prevaccination era. No lead was uncovered by testing paired sera from pediatric patients with unidentified viral infections, or sera obtained during prospective studies of viral infections done by Henle et al. (1968). The key clue to the illness associated with this virus arose unexpectedly when their technician, E.H., developed infectious mononucleosis. Her serum, which lacked EBV anti-

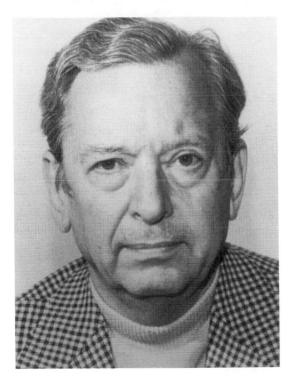

Figure 3.6.   Werner Henle, 1910–1986, Chief, Virology Laboratory, Children's Hospital, University of Pennsylvania (from Evans, 1976).

body prior to illness, developed EBV-IgC antibody to the viral capsid antigen (VCA) in a titer of 1:40 during the illness. Her leukocytes, which could not be grown in culture prior to illness, now grew well within 4 weeks, and 4 weeks later were shown to harbor EBV antigen. This observation led to a study in which all of 42 Yale students with acute infectious mononucleosis were found to have EBV antibody, whereas of 50 sera randomly selected from healthy Yale controls, only 24% had antibody (Niederman *et al.*, 1968). They also showed that EBV antibody was absent in preillness sera from 12 patients who later developed infectious mononucleosis, and was accompanied by the appearance of antibody during illness. These findings have now been amply confirmed in prospective cohort studies carried out on Yale University students (Evans *et al.*, 1968; Niederman *et al.*, 1971; Sawyer *et al.*, 1971), on cadets at the West Point Military Academy (Hallee *et al.*, 1974), and in several English colleges and universities (University Health Physicians, 1971). The accumulated evidence from 3,243 students indicated that antibody to EBV is regularly absent prior to illness and regularly appears during clinical infectious mononucleosis. The absence of this antibody at the start of the prospective observation period is a reliable indicator of susceptibility to EBV infection and to clinical infectious mononucleosis, and the presence of antibody is a reliable indicator of immunity to both infection and the disease. The consistency and longitudinal nature of the epidemiological data established, on immunological grounds alone, that EBV was beyond a reasonable doubt the single cause of heterophile positive infectious mononucleosis (Evans, 1974). It was also shown that both EBV and, to a much smaller extent, cytomegalovirus (Evans, 1978) could cause a similar syndrome lacking heterophile antibody. Later technical developments demonstrated that in the laboratory, the virus could infect B lymphocytes present in the cord blood of infants and of adults lacking EBV antibody. With the use of this method, EB viral excretion was demonstrated in the throat in about 80% of patients during the acute stage of the illness and persisted intermittently in the throat in some 15– 20% of infected persons over several years, if not for life. The presence of EBV was also shown in lymphocytes cultured from the blood, where it also persists in latent form over one's lifetime. Current data are still inadequate to fulfill the Henle–Koch postulates, since the agent is present in healthy carriers and has not been isolated in pure culture, and the disease has not been fully "reproduced anew" experimentally. For these reasons, a new set of guidelines of causation based on immunological criteria was proposed, as shown in Table 3.5. These criteria have been fulfilled for EBV as a cause of infectious mononucleosis, and may also be applicable to other situations in which the causative agent cannot be grown in the laboratory, or in which a susceptible experimental animal cannot be found. A sixth and final criterion to be fulfilled after the agent has been isolated and grown in pure culture is that "production of antibody to the agent (immunization) should prevent the disease, or at least that portion of the syndrome

Table 3.5
Elements of Immunological Proof of Causation[a]

1.	Antibody to the agent is regularly absent prior to the disease and to exposure to the agent (i.e., before the incubation period).
2.	Antibody to the agent regularly appears during illness and includes both IgG- and IgM-type antibodies.
3.	The presence of antibody to the agent indicates immunity to the clinical disease associated with primary infection by the agent.
4.	The absence of antibody to the agent indicates susceptibility to both infection and the disease produced by the agent.
5.	Antibody to no other agent should be similarly associated with the disease unless it is a cofactor in its production.

[a]Derived from Evans (1976).

attributable to that agent." This has not yet been shown for infectious mono-nucleosis, although Epstein and his group, as well as others, have prepared vaccines that are nearly ready to test in humans (Epstein, 1986, 1990).

New Diseases

Acquired Immunodeficiency Syndrome (AIDS)

Official recognition of AIDS, currently a worldwide epidemic, began on June 5, 1981, with an item in the *Morbidity and Mortality Weekly Reports* (MMWR) of the Centers for Disease Control (CDC) regarding five cases of *Pneumocystis* pneumonia in males, age 29–36, all homosexuals, living in the city of Los Angeles (Centers for Disease Control, 1981a). The five men did not know one another; all had used inhalant drugs, one parenteral drugs; and four were hepatitis B antigen positive. This disease ordinarily occurs in older persons with cancer and an immunocompromised immune system and had almost never before been seen in the United States in previously healthy persons. The CDC received early notification because it controlled the distribution of pentamidine, one of the drugs used in the treatment of pneumonia. This report was followed on July 3, 1981 with the report of *Pneumocystis* pneumonia and/or of Kaposi's sarcoma in 41 male homosexuals in New York City or California (Centers for Disease Control, 1981b). Actually, such cases had been recognized by physicians in both New York City and California in the late 1970s, but the epidemic character of the illness was not yet recognized. Eventually, however, case reports continued to increase, the clinical spectrum was enlarged, and the groups at highest risk were identified. This early history is recorded up to May 1983 (Evans, 1984) in Figure 3.7. The clinical spectrum included a group of symptoms due to infectious agents, many of which were not ordinarily pathogenic in healthy humans: *Pneumocystis carinii,* cryptosporidiosis, *Mycobacterium avium intracellulare,* and several fungi, diseases of the central nervous system associated with the reactivation of latent agents (toxoplasmosis, coccidiodomycosis, progressive focal leukoencephalopathy from papovavirus, and various types of meningoencephalitis due to cytomegalovirus and other agents). In addition to Kaposi's sarcoma, several types of lymphoma were observed. EBV was later recognized in all lymphomas of the brain, and in about one-third of non-Hodgkins lymphomas and several malignancies closely associated with reactivated viral agents occurring in AIDS patients (Biggar and Rabkin, in press). Later, after the inciting agent, HIV, was identified, an early mono-like syndrome was described (Kessler *et al.,* 1987) and a direct involvement of the central nervous system, termed HIV encephalopathy or dementia complex were noted (Price *et al.,* 1988). Both of these were direct effects of the virus rather than an indirect result of an impaired immune system. The four major risk groups described initially were male homosexuals (71%), I.V. drug users (17%), Haitians (5%), and hemophiliacs (6%). The association with Haitians was later found to be unrelated to ethnic origin and more probably due to male prostitution and reuse of unsterilized needles by native practitioners in Haiti; the designation as a risk group was then dropped. The relation to hemophilia was recognized as due to contamination of Factor VIII of blood used in therapy that had been contaminated by blood donated by homosexuals and I.V. drug users infected with the infectious agent. The occurrence of AIDS in transfused infants, in female sex partners of AIDS patients, the recognition of asymptomatic male carriers, and the presence of the disease in at least 16 other countries had all been recognized by May 1983 (Centers for Disease Control, 1983). Intensive epidemiological, clinical, immunological, microbiological, and pathological studies were initiated by many investigators, including those at the National Institutes of Health (NIH), especially at the National Cancer Institute, and at the CDC. The key immunological finding was of a defect in the immune system characterized by a reversal of the T4/T8 lymphocyte ratio below 1.0, due primarily to a reduction in T4 lymphocytes. Because no etiologic agent could be isolated despite vigorous investigation, the CDC was forced to adopt a working definition, as they had done for Legionnaire's disease, which described certain key immunological and clinical features, as they were known at the time (Centers for Disease Control, 1982). The main points in the definition were that a previously healthy adult under the age of 60 years and with no known cause of immunosuppression develops a clinical disease that is predictive of a defect in cellular immune function, such as those mentioned above. Case–control studies launched by the

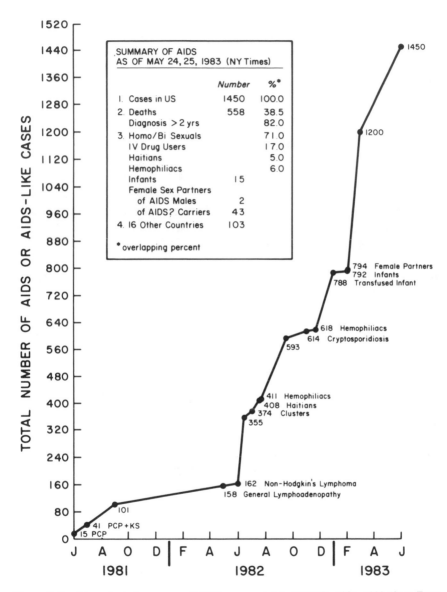

Figure 3.7. Chronological sequence of AIDS as reported in MMWR, 1981–1983 (from Evans, 1984).

CDC compared various features of 50 patients that fulfilled CDC's definition with 120 control homosexuals (78 from a clinic and 42 from private practice) (Jaffe *et al.*, 1983). The variable most strongly associated with illness was a larger number of male sex partners per year in AIDS patients (median 61) as compared with 27 in private practice and 25 in clinic controls. In addition, cases were more likely than controls to have been exposed to feces during sex, have had syphilis or non-B hepatitis, have been treated for enteric diseases, and have used various illicit substances. A companion paper reported the laboratory results in these groups (Rogers *et al.*, 1983). No etiological agent was isolated but patients were found to have lymphopenia, specifically a deficiency in the helper T cell (T4) population, a reversal of the T4/T8 (suppressor) ratio, increased levels of IgG and IgA, higher antibody titers to EBV and cytomegalovirus (CMV), a higher prevalence of antibody to hepatitis A virus and *Treponema pallidum,* and a higher frequency of isolation of CMV. Other investigators were obtaining similar results. Many hypotheses of pathogenesis and etiology were proposed but most investigators grew to suspect an infectious origin with CMV, EBV, and HBV being named as candidate agents. In March 1983, Gellman and Gallo of the National Cancer Institute suggested the retroviruses as the possible cause at a meeting in New York City (Gellmann *et al.*, 1983). In May of the same year, four papers appeared in *Science* from Montagnier's group (Figure 3.8) at the Pasteur Institute in Paris (Barre-Sinoussi *et al.*, 1983), from Gallo (Figure 3.9) and his group, and from Essex *et al.* at the Harvard School of Public Health (Essex *et al.*, 1983), all suggesting that a retrovirus termed human T-cell leuke-mia virus (HTLV) by the NIH team and lymphadenopathy virus (LAV) by the French team was closely associated with AIDS (Research News, 1983). Unfortu-nately, the virus could be isolated from only 3 of 35 AIDS patients studied by Gallo and associates (Gallo *et al.*, 1983) and antibody to the cell membrane of the virus could be demonstrated, often in low titer, in only 25.3% of AIDS patients and in 26% of patients with the lymphadenopathy syndrome, as com-pared with one of 71 matched controls and none of 139 blood donors (Essex *et al.*, 1983). In September 1983, a conference on the "Epidemiology of AIDS" was held at the NIH at which I proposed that a prospective serological study be carried out to identify the possible etiological agent using HTLV, EBV, CMV, and HBV as prime markers (Evans, 1983). I estimated that about half of active homosexuals would be "susceptible" as indicated by a normal T4/T8 ratio, the absence of HTLV antibody, and normal levels of EBV and CMV antibodies. I estimated that 10% would become infected with HTLV yearly and that 2–10% of these would develop clinical manifestations of AIDS. After long delays in being accepted, this paper was subsequently published along with a hypothesis on the pathogenesis of AIDS involving the consequences of a T-cell cascade initiated by infection of T4 cells with an HTLV-like virus, and by a B-cell cascade initiated by the reactivation of EBV in lymphocytes leading to a polyclonal B-cell pro-liferation and the appearance of B-cell lymphomas (Evans, 1984). The low

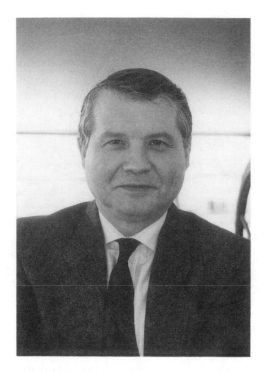

Figure 3.8. Dr. Luc Montagnier, 1932– , Chief, Viral Oncology Unit, Pasteur Institute, Paris, France.

isolation rate of HTLV, type I from patients (about 8%) and the low frequency of antibody responses in AIDS and lymphadenopathy patients (about 25%) cast doubt that this virus was the exact strain producing the disease or that the sensitivity of the tests used for isolation and antibody testing were very poor. The real breakthrough came when the French team headed by Montagnier isolated a related retrovirus called lymphadenopathy virus (LAV) by them (Villmer *et al.*, 1984) and the NIH team headed by Gallo announced the isolation and serological evidence favoring a new retrovirus termed HTLV, type III (HTLV-III), in four papers in *Science* in May 1984 (Popovic *et al.*, 1984; Gallo *et al.*, 1984; Schupbach *et al.*, 1984; Sarngadharan *et al.*, 1984). Both agents are now known to be identical, and termed the human immunodeficiency virus (HIV) by an international committee. An excellent editorial by Marx in the same issue of *Science* summarized the strong evidence that this virus was the cause of AIDS (Marx, 1984). This evidence was based on case–control isolation and antibody studies as summarized in Table 3.6. The relatively low isolation rate from patients is probably due to the loss of infected T4 cells by lysis from the virus, leaving too few for isolation procedures, or to a lack of sensitivity of the isolation methods.

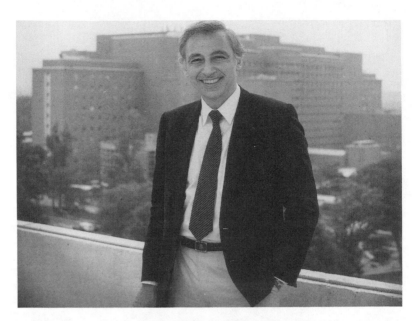

Figure 3.9.   Dr. Robert Gallo, 1937– , Chief, Laboratory of Tumor Cell Biology, National Cancer Institute, National Institutes of Health, Bethesda, Maryland.

Prospective studies have now been carried out in a multicenter cohort investigation showing that 8% of susceptible male homosexuals became infected with HIV (I will now use this term rather than HTLV-III or LAV) over a 2-year period, as demonstrated by the appearance of HIV-specific antibody, and the development of clinical AIDS in much of this group. The highest rate of infection was in those practicing receptive anal intercourse, and no infection occurred among 220 homosexuals who did not practice any type of anal intercourse. The rate of *clinical disease* among 1835 HIV-infected homosexuals was 3.2% over 15 months. Other follow-up studies of HIV-antibody–positive persons over 5–7 years have shown a 30–50% rate of AIDS, more with AIDS-related complex, and others with CNS manifestations or malignancies; only 20% remained asymptomatic (Curran *et al.*, 1988). The inoculation of HIV into experimental animals has not yet reproduced the clinical picture of AIDS, although nonhuman primates have been infected in the laboratory and a simian-AIDS virus produces a similar disease in nature. Very sensitive enzyme-linked immunosorbent assay (ELISA) tests for antibody have now been developed permitting screening of blood donors and use as a diagnostic test. Less than 5% false positives occur in approved laboratories and a highly specific antibody technique called Western blot has been used to separate out the true positives. There is also a false-negative rate of about 5% in patients who have demonstrable circulating virus but no detectable antibody, either because it has not developed yet, fails to develop in immunosuppressed individuals, or is in too low titer to be detected by the test. The presence of HIV antigenemia has now been demonstrated in many such persons prior to the appearance of antibody. For example, Phair (1987) found antigen in 51 of 71 seronegative homosexuals who subsequently developed AIDS. The polymerase chain reaction (PCR) is now widely used to demonstrate HIV antigen in blood and tissues (Poiesz *et al.*, 1990).

Table 3.6
AIDS, April 1990[a]

	Approximate Figures	
United States	1988	1992 (estimated)
New cases	30,000	80,000
Cumulative cases	133,889	365,000
Cumulative deaths	50%	263,000

About 10% of all deaths in ages 25–44 are due to AIDS

Estimated number of HIV-infected persons in U.S.: 1–1.5 million
Percentage of HIV-infected I.V. drug users in certain areas:

Washington, D.C.	28%
Los Angeles and Seattle	5%
New York	50%
New Jersey	12–43%

Pattern: Changing from homosexual to greater percentage in I.V. drug users, their sexual partners and their children (1000 now with 84% in blacks and Hispanics)

Worldwide—1988

Total cumulative cases	377,000	
Africa	200,000	(mostly heterosexuals)
North America	110,000	
Latin America	40,000	
Europe	25,000	
Aust., New Zeal., Pac.	1,500	
Asia	500	

Total infected: about 5 million

[a]From: *MMWR* **38** (suppl 4) May 12, 1989 and **38**:793, November 24, 1989.

By August 1985, the epidemic reached worldwide proportions with an estimated 1 million persons infected in the United States, and by mid-1988 this had risen to 1.5–2.0 million estimated to be infected and over 60,000 cases had been reported to the CDC. By 1992, over 200,000 cases and over 100,000 deaths were recorded. About half of the infected cases have died and the final mortality of AIDS approaches 100%. Many prevalence studies for HIV antibody have now been carried out throughout many parts of the world as summarized by Gutensohn (personal communication, 1985). Among homosexuals in six large U.S. cities, the prevalence rates in 1984 varied from 28 to 68%. In a cohort study of 6875 homosexuals carried out by the CDC (Echenberg *et al.*, 1985) over a 7-year period in San Francisco with antibody testing in 1978, 1980, and 1984, the prevalence rate rose from 4% in 1978 to 68% in 1984, and the estimated average increase in prevalence rate was 10.3%, close to my 1983 estimate (Evans, 1983). Of 4675 homosexuals positive for antibody over this period, 188 or 4.0% have thus far developed clinical AIDS. Given an average incubation period of about 5–7 years, the final clinical rate may be several times this. Canadian cities have shown a little lower prevalence with 28% in Vancouver and in Montreal.

In homosexual men in Europe, antibody prevalence rates in 1984 were 49% in Sweden, 35% in West Germany, 22–35% in three studies in England, 30% in Rome, 18% in Switzerland, and 0% in Hungary (Gutensohn, personal communication, 1985). AIDS has now been recognized in Russia as well as Australia and Japan. In Africa, children and adults have been shown to have varying antibody prevalence rates for both HTLV-I and HIV antibody in different geographic areas and in different risk groups. In Rwanda, prostitutes had HTLV-III prevalence rates of 81%, their customers 28%, blood donors 19%, and maternity patients 5%; in Zaire rates of 12% and in Kenya 6–51% have been reported (Gutensohn, personal communication, 1985). In the West Nile district of Uganda, 50 of 75 sera collected prior to 1973 were positive and 12 of these were also positive for HTLV-I antibody (Biggar *et al.*, 1984).

Up to 80% of some African population groups have been positive in some areas (Biggar *et al.*, 1984) but strangely enough with very few cases of reported AIDS. Whether this was due to failure to recognize the disease, to a relatively avirulent strain of virus that results in few clinical manifestations, to a more benign course when the virus is not introduced in a traumatized rectum or intravenously, or to the young age of the subjects at the time of infection is not currently known. In a more recent update on the international status, as of December 1988, Piot and associates at the World Health Organization (Piot *et al.*, 1988) stated that 8652 cases had been reported to them from Africa. In addition, 55,354 had been reported from the Americas, 224 from Asia, 8775 from Europe, and 742 from Oceania, a grand total of 73,747. An update as of June 1991 covering the first 10 years is given in Table 3.7.

At the present time, the virus has been demonstrated in the blood, especially

Table 3.7
HIV/AIDS: The First Ten Years[a]

In the United States
   Total cases reported since 1981   179,136
   Total deaths (63%)   >113,000

   Leading cause of death of:
     Men and women under 45 years old
     Children under 5 years old

   Male 87.9% Female   12.1%
   White 51.6% Black   30.4% Hispanic 16.9%

   Age 20–29, 19.2%; 30–39, 45.5%; 40–49, 23.1%

   Transmission
     Male homo/bisexuals   54.8%
     IV drug users
       Women and heterosexual men   23.1%
       Male homo/bisexuals   5.3%
     Hemophiliacs   0.9%
     Transfusion recipients   2.1%

In the world
  Now:
    Estimated number of adults infected: 8–10 million
    Estimated number of children infected: 1 million
  By year 2000:
    Estimated number infected: 40 million
    (90% of these will reside in developing areas)

[a]From *MMWR* **40:**357 (June 7), 1991.

in T4 lymphocytes, but also free in various blood fractions, as well as in mono-cytes, macrophages, cells of the central nervous system, lung tissue, and rectal epithelium. Some of these cells bear the same CD4 receptor for HIV as do T4 lymphocytes (Fauci, 1988). In some, the virus is cytocidal and in others it is not. The virus is present in genital secretions, in semen, in saliva, and in tears. The major routes of transmission are by sexual intercourse, both homosexual and heterosexual (at a lower rate and with more efficient transmission from males to females), by blood transfusions and use of other blood products contaminated by the virus, and by intravenous drug users. The virus may pass from infected mother to infant either during pregnancy, during delivery, or subsequently. Most infections are probably acquired during passage through the birth canal. Pediatric AIDS is becoming a very important problem but has a shorter incubation period and rather different clinical manifestations than in adults, such as lymphocytic interstitial pneumonitis in association with EBV. No evidence of person-to-person transmission has been shown in careful family and contact studies (Curran *et al.,* 1988) and an extremely low risk is associated with health care personnel taking care of AIDS patients. The major danger lies in sticking oneself with a needle contaminated with HIV from a patient, a risk estimated to be about 1 in 200. Since HIV infection is often symptomatic, all hospital and clinic patients must be regarded as potentially infected and "universal precautions" taken by all health personnel (Centers for Disease Control, 1987). The epidemiology of HIV infection closely resembles that of hepatitis B virus, which can be transmitted in children in long, close, institutional settings and among family members, and despite the much lower infectivity of HIV, I am still concerned about its transmission over time in a mixture of infected and uninfected children in long intimate contact, especially in retarded children and with biting and scratching going on. This has not occurred to date but its potential raises critical issues about admission to school, to day-care centers, and in young adults to the armed forces and to colleges, especially when an antibody test can detect present or past infection without knowledge of the consequences of this finding. The protection of human rights and of civil liberties conflict in these settings with the public health issue of identifying the infected and protecting the uninfected from any possible routes of spread. It is my guess that HIV antibody testing, now required in the armed forces and other sensitive government posts, will become more widespread, especially as economic issues, such as health care insurance in big insurance companies and big industries, conflict with the human rights issue. The same moral issues pertained to syphilis earlier in the century, but syphilis is rarely fatal, and is a treatable disease. The growing impact of this great epidemic on the health and economy of humankind may make the identification of HIV-infected persons and the prevention of spread to others a more compelling issue than issues of confidentiality and civil rights.

    The important issue from the standpoint of this book is: Does HIV cause AIDS? In my view it does not directly produce the symptoms of AIDS, as defined by the original definition of the CDC, but does directly result in an early mono-like illness and HIV encephalopathy that were not part of the original definition of AIDS (Centers for Disease Control, 1982). HIV produces an altered state of lowered susceptibility in the human host through destruction of T4 lymphocytes, but by itself, does not produce the clinical disease defined as AIDS. This syndrome is due to various external or commensal organisms, often of low or absent pathogenicity in the healthy host, and by the reactivation of many viral, bacterial, and fungal agents. It is really an almost unique situation in infectious diseases. Many other infectious agents may require cofactors within or without the host to result in illness but the disease consequences are usually a direct result of the effect of the agent or of an immunological response induced by it. As discussed later, the effect of a microbial agent on tissues may be a direct lytic one or operate through various immunological mechanisms, but whatever the mechanism, the infectious agent is intimately involved in the pathogenetic process. In the same vein, one might ask if renal transplantation with its attendant drug-induced immunosuppression is "the cause" of the various infectious and malignant diseases that may follow in the wake of this procedure. Or does Hodgkin's disease cause progressive multifocal leukoencephalopathy (PML) because it reactivates the papovavirus that leads to the disease in about 80% of the PML cases? HIV appears to be a necessary but insufficient "cause" of the syndromes that follow in its wake. It is also likely that, if an effective vaccine can be developed, AIDS could be prevented. This demonstration would be a very strong argument for a causal relationship between a suspected agent and a disease. While the control of AIDS seems very difficult at present, and a vaccine would seem to be the most important approach, difficulty is being encountered in the production of enough virus and in identifying a common antigenic protein in the variations encountered in the strains of HIV thus far tested. From a causal viewpoint, it is obvious that the problem is largely semantic as to what the cause–effect relationship should mean in a pathogenetic sense.

The above view of HIV causation was written in August 1985, except for the addition of the mono-like syndrome and CNS involvement described since then. In October 1987, Professor Peter Duesberg (Figure 3.10), a distinguished molecular virologist at the University of California, Berkeley, expressed similar views in a well-documented article that also expressed his view of the limited role of retroviruses in oncogenesis (Duesberg, 1987). These views on HIV have been more recently restated (Duesberg, 1988) in an article entitled "HIV Does Not Cause AIDS." His view appears to be that neither retroviruses nor HIV are necessary or sufficient to produce cancer or AIDS respectively, and that neither fulfill the Henle–Koch postulates. His opinions have created much angry and vigorous reaction in the scientific community, including leading AIDS researchers (Booth, 1988a,b; Fauci, 1988), and have been responded to in a brief discussion of Duesberg's article in *Science* (1988) by Blattner *et al.* (1988) and in AIDS by Ginzberg *et al.* (1988). I agree with Duesberg that HIV is not the single, *necessary* cause of AIDS as infection with another virus, HIV-2, has been shown to result in AIDS in Africa (Clavel *et al.*, 1986). I also agree that HIV is not a *sufficient* cause since it is dependent on the presence of other latent and/or opportunistic organisms to result in the clinical features. I also agree that HIV does not fulfill the Henle–Koch postulates, but as pointed out earlier in this chapter, few viruses do fulfill them, and none, if "pure culture" means bacterial

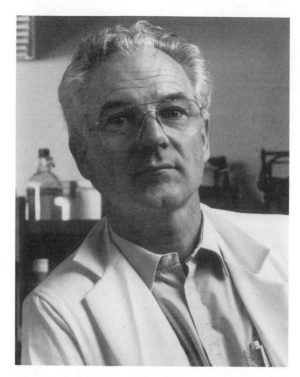

Figure 3.10. Dr. Peter Duesberg, 1936– , Professor of Molecular and Cell Biology, University of California, Berkeley (by permission of photographer Robert Holmgren).

culture, as outlined by Rivers (1937) and Huebner (1957). However, I strongly disagree with Duesberg's statement that "since the cause of AIDS is debatable, the control of AIDS may not be achieved by controlling HIV." I think that nothing should deter us from the control of the transmission of HIV, from work toward the development of a vaccine, and from the search for antiviral or immunological techniques to prevent the development of AIDS among those infected. If these can be accomplished, then that percentage of AIDS attributable to the consequences of HIV infection would sharply decrease, and be strong evidence of its role in the pathogenesis of the syndrome. A small percentage due to HIV-2 or even HTLV-I would not be reduced by a specific vaccine but would be by control of similar routes of transmission. Philosophical arguments on semantic issues in causation should not deter us from this task. I also disagree with much of the evidence given by Duesberg in his original paper (1987), or at least, his interpretations of the evidence. However, I have responded to these in detail elsewhere (Evans, 1989a,b,c). Duesberg has reviewed my arguments and believes we are in agreement on six points and disagree on two (Duesberg, 1989), to which I responded that the two points on which we disagreed were critical ones (Evans, 1989b). One was that I believed that HIV led to AIDS, and the other was that our public policy was, and should be, directed at the spread of this virus. Duesberg has remained unconvinced and continues to express his view that HIV has nothing to do with AIDS (Duesberg, 1991), based in part on the failure of HIV to fulfill the Koch postulates, now one hundred years old. I replied that these postulates have many limitations, some recognized by Koch himself, and that Duesberg should follow the modern guidelines of causal proof that incorporate our newer concepts of epidemiology and pathogenesis (Evans, 1992).

References

Barre-Sinoussi F, Chermann JC, Rey F, *et al:* Isolation of T lymphotropi retrovirus from a patient at risk for acquired immunodeficiency syndrome (AIDS). *Science* **220:**868–871, 1983.

Biggar RJ, Saxinger C, Gardiner C, *et al:* Type-1 HTLV antibody in urban and rural Ghana, West Africa. *Int J Cancer* **34:**215–219, 1984.

Blattner W, Gallo RC, Temin HM, *et al:* Blattner and colleagues respond to Duesberg. *Science* **241:**514–515, 1988.

Blumberg BS, Alter HJ, Riddell NM, *et al:* Multiple antigenic specificities of serum lipoproteins detected with sera of transfused patients. *Vox Sang* **9:**128–145, 1964.

Blumberg BS, Alter HJ, Visnich S: A 'new' antigen in leukemia sera. *JAMA* **191:**541–546, 1965.

Blumberg BS, Gerstley BJ, Hungerford DA, *et al:* A serum antigen (Australia antigen) in Down's syndrome, leukemia and hepatitis. *Ann Intern Med* **66:**924–931, 1967.

Booth W: A rebel without a cause. *Science* **239:**1485–1488, 1988a.

Booth W: Duesberg gets his day in court. *Science* **240:**279, 1988b.

Burkitt DP: A sarcoma involving the jaws in African children. *Br J Surg* **46:**218–223, 1958.

Centers for Disease Control: *Pneumocystis* pneumonia—Los Angeles. *MMWR* **30:**250–252, 1981a.

Centers for Disease Control: Kaposi's sarcoma and *Pneumocystis* pneumonia among homosexual men—New York City and California. *MMWR* **30:**305–308, 1981b.

Centers for Disease Control: Update on acquired immune deficiency syndrome (AIDS) in the United States. *MMWR* **31:**505–508, 513, 593, 1982.

Centers for Disease Control: Update. Acquired immunodeficiency syndrome (AIDS)—United States. *MMWR* **32:**465–467, 1983a.

Centers for Disease Control: Human T-cell leukemia virus infection in patients with acquired immunodeficiency syndrome: Preliminary observations. *MMWR* **32:**233–234, 1983b.

Centers for Disease Control: Recommendations for prevention of HIV transmission in health-care settings. *MMWR* **36**(Suppl.) 3S–128S, 1987.

Centers for Disease Control: HIV/AIDS. The first ten years. *MMWR* **40:**357, 1991.

Clavel F, Guetard D, Brun-Vazinet, *et al:* Isolation of a new human retrovirus from West African patients with AIDS. *Science* **233:**343–346, 1986.

Curran JW, Jaffe HW, Hardy A, *et al:* Epidemiology of HIV infection and AIDS in the United States. *Science* **239:**610–616, 1988.

Duesburg P: Retrovirus as carcinogens and pathogens. Expectations and reality. *Cancer Res* **47:**1199–1226, 1987.

Duesburg P: HIV is not the cause of AIDS. *Science* **241:**514–516, 1988.

Duesburg P: Does HIV cause AIDS? (Letter to the editor.) *J Acq Immunodef Dis* **2:**514–517, 1989.

Duesburg P: AIDS epidemiology. Inconsistencies with human immunodeficiency virus and with infectious disease. *Proc Natl Acad Sci USA* **88:**1575–1579, 1991.

Echenberg DF, Rutherford G, O'Malley P, *et al:* Update: Acquired immunodeficiency syndrome in the San Francisco cohort study, 1978–1985. *MMWR* **34:**573–575, 1985.

Epstein MA: Vaccination against Epstein–Barr virus: Current progress and future strategies. *Lancet* **1:**1425–1427, 1986.

Epstein MA: Plans for human trials of a vaccine against Epstein–Barr virus infection, in La Maza LM, Peterson EM (eds): *Medical Virology.* New York, Plenum Press, 1990, vol 9, pp 207–216.

Epstein MA, Achong BG, Barr YM: Virus particles in cultured lymphoblasts from Burkitt lymphoma. *Lancet* **1:**702–703, 1964.

Essex M, McLane, Lee TH, *et al:* Antibodies to cell membrane antigens associated with human T-cell leukemia virus in patients with AIDS. *Science* **220:**850–862, 1983.

Evans AS: Clinical syndromes in adults caused by respiratory infection. *Med Clin North Am* **51:**803–815, 1967.

Evans AS: New discoveries in infectious mononucleosis. *Mod Med* **42:**18–24, 1974.

Evans AS: Infectious mononucleosis and related syndromes. *Am J Med Sci* **276:**325–339, 1978.

Evans AS: Causation and disease. The Henle-Koch postulates revisited. *Yale J Biol Med* **49:**175–195, 1976.

Evans AS: Prospective seroepidemiologial studies. Applications to studies of AIDS. Presented at NIH workshop on epidemiology of AIDS, Bethesda, Maryland, September 11–13, 1984.

Evans AS: Hypothesis: The pathogenesis of AIDS. Activation of the T- and B-cell cascades. *Yale J Biol Med* **57:**317–327, 1984.

Evans AS: Author's reply to letter from Duesberg on "Does HIV cause AIDS?" *J AIDS* **2:**515–517, 1989a.

Evans AS: Does HIV cause AIDS? An historical perspective. *J AIDS* **2:**107–113, 1989b.

Evans AS (ed): *Viral Infections of Humans: Epidemiology and Control,* 3rd ed. New York, Plenum Press, 1989c.

Evans AS: AIDS: The alternative view. *Lancet* **339:**1547, 1992.

Evans AS, Niederman JC, McCollum RW: Seroepidemiological studies of infectious mononucleosis with EB virus. *N Engl J Med* **279:**1121–1127, 1968.

Fauci AS: The human immunodeficiency virus: Infectivity and mechanisms of pathogenesis. *Science* **239:**617–622, 1988.

Fox JP, Hall CP: *Surveillance of Families as a Key to Epidemiology of Virus Infections.* Littleton, MA, PSG Publishing Co, 1980.

Gallo R, Sarin PS, Gellmann EP, *et al:* Isolation of human T cell leukemia virus in acquired immune deficiency syndrome (AIDS). *Science* **220:**865–866, 1983.

Gallo RO, Salahuddin SC, Papovic M, *et al:* Frequent detection and isolation of cytopathic retroviruses (HTLV-III) from patients with AIDS and at high risk for AIDS. *Science* **224:**500–502, 1989.

Gellmann E, Gallo R: A search for retroviruses in patients with diseases associated with the acquired immune deficiency. Presented at the conference on epidemic Kaposi's sarcoma and opportunistic infections in homosexual men: Expression of an acquired immunoregulatory disorder, New York University, March 17–19, 1983.

Giles JP, McCollum RW, Berndtson LW Jr, *et al:* Relation of Australia-SH antigen to the Willowbrook MS-2 strain. *N Engl J Med* **28:**19–22, 1969.

Ginzberg HM, Fleming PL, Miller KD: Selected public health observations from the multicenter AIDS cohort study. *J AIDS* **1:**2–7, 1988.

Gutensohn N: Personal communication, 1985.

Hallee TJ, Evans AS, Niederman JC, *et al:* Infectious mononucleosis at the U.S. Military Academy: A prospective study of a single class over four years. *Yale J Biol Med* **47:**182–195, 1974.

Henle G, Henle W: Immunofluorescence in cells derived from Burkitt's lymphoma. *J Bacteriol* **91**:1248–1256, 1966.

Henle G, Henle W, Diehl V: Relation of Burkitt's tumor-associated virus to infectious mononucleosis. *Proc Natl Acad Sci USA* **59**:94–101, 1968.

Huebner RJ: The virologist's dilemma. *Ann NY Acad Sci* **67**:430–442, 1957.

Jaffe HW, Keewhan C, Thomas P, *et al:* National case–control study of Kaposi's sarcoma and *Pneumocystis carinii* pneumonia in homosexual men. Part 1. Epidemiologic results. *Ann Intern Med* **99**:145–151, 1983.

Kessler HA, Blaovir B, Spear J, *et al:* Diagnosis of human immunodeficiency virus infection in seronegative homosexuals presenting with an acute viral syndrome. *JAMA* **258**:1196–1199, 1987.

Krugman S, Giles JP, Hammond J: Infectious hepatitis: Evidence for two distinctive clinical, epidemiological, and immunological types of infection. *JAMA* **200**:95–103, 1967.

Krugman S, Giles JP, Hammond J: Hepatis virus: Effect of heat on the infectivity and antigenicity of the MS-1 and MS-2 strain. *J Infect Dis* **122**:423–436, 1970.

Marx JL: Strong new candidate for AIDS agent. A newly discovered member of the human T-cell leukemia virus family is very closely linked to the immunodeficiency disease. *Science* **224**:475–477, 1984.

McCollum RW: Viral hepatitis, in Evans AS (ed): *Viral Infections of Humans: Epidemiology and Control,* 2nd ed. New York, Plenum Press, 1982, pp 327–350.

Niederman JC, McCollum RW, Henle G, *et al:* Infectious mononucleosis: Clinical manifestations in relation to EB virus antibodies. *JAMA* **203**:200–209, 1968.

Okoche K, Murakami S: Observations on Australia antigen in Japanese. *Vox Sang* **15**:374–385, 1968.

Phair HP: Editorial. Human immunodeficiency virus antigenemia. *JAMA* **258**:1218, 1987.

Piot P, Plummer FA, Mhalu FS, *et al:* AIDS: An international perspective. *Science* **239**:573–579, 1988.

Poiesz BJ, Erlich GD, Byrne BC, *et al:* The use of the polymerase chain reaction in the detection, quantitation, and characterization of human retroviruses, in de la Mesa LM, Peterson, EM (eds): *Medical Virology.* New York, Plenum Press, 1990, vol 9, pp 47–76.

Popovic M, Sarngadharan MG, Read E, *et al:* Detection, isolation and continuous production of cytopathic retroviruses (HTLV-III) from patients with AIDS and pre-AIDS. *Science* **224**:497–500, 1984.

Price RV, Brew B, Sidtis J, *et al:* The brain in AIDS. Central nervous system symptoms of HIV-1 infection and AIDS dementia complex. *Science* **239**:586–592, 1988.

Prince AM: An antigen detected in the blood during the incubation period of serum hepatitis. *Proc Natl Acad Sci USA* **60**:814–821, 1968.

Robkin CS, Biggar RJ, Horn JW: Increasing incidence of cancer associated with human immunodeficiency virus outbreak. *Int J Cancer* **12**:692–696, 1991.

Research news: Human T cell leukemia virus linked to AIDS. *Science* **220**:806–807, 1983.

Rivers TM: Viruses and Koch's postulates. *J Bacteriol* **33**:1–12, 1937.

Rivers TM, Horsfall FL (eds): *Viral and Rickettsial Infections of Man,* 3rd ed. New York, J B Lippincott Co, 1959.

Rogers MF, Morens DW, Stewart JA, *et al:* National case–control study of Kaposi's sarcoma and *Pneumocystis carinii* pneumonia in homosexual men. Part 2. Laboratory results. *Ann Intern Med* **99**:151–158, 1983.

Sarngadharan MG, Popovic M, Bruch, L, *et al:* Antibodies reactive with human T-lymphotrophic retroviruses (HTLV-III) in the serum of patients with AIDS. *Science* **224**:506–508, 1984.

Sawyer RN, Evans AS, McCollum RW: Prospective studies of a group of Yale University freshmen. 1. Occurrence of infectious mononucleosis. *J Infect Dis* **123**:263–269, 1971.

Schupbach J, Popovic M, Gilden RV, *et al:* Serological analysis of a subgroup of human T-cell lymphotrophic retroviruses (HTLV-III) associated with AIDS. *Science* **224:**503–505, 1984.

Shope RE: Swine influenza III. Filtration experiments and etiology. *J Exp Med* **54:**373–385, 1931.

Szmuness W, Stevens CE, Harley EJ, *et al:* Hepatitis B vaccine. Demonstration of efficacy in a controlled clinical trial in a high risk population in the United States. *N Engl J Med* **303:**833–841, 1973.

University Health Physicians and P.H.L.S. Laboratories. A joint investigation. Infectious mononucleosis and its relationship to EB virus antibody. *Br Med J* **4:**643–646, 1971.

Villmer E, Barre-Sinoussi F, Rouzioux C, *et al:* Isolation of a new lymphotropic retrovirus from two patients with hemophilia B, one with AIDS. *Lancet* **1:**753–757, 1984.

Slow and Persistent Viral Infections

Introduction

There are two types of viral infections that bring about chronic, progressive, and usually fatal diseases involving the central nervous system (CNS). Each of them poses problems in meeting the postulates of causation thus far discussed. One type is caused by a unique group of viruses with no detectable immune response. These viruses are called "slow viruses" or "lentiviruses" because of the long period between exposure and the appearance of clinical disease, which presumably reflects the primary incubation or multiplication time for the agents. The second type of infection is caused by a group of several common and ubiquitous viruses that affect the brain several years after the primary infection and that are associated with an aberrant immune response. The two groups will be discussed separately because they require different criteria to establish a causal relationship between the virus and the disease. Certain members of the retrovirus family that bear a molecular resemblance to some of the slow viruses of animals are suspected of causing chronic infections of the CNS in humans. There are also several chronic and progressive diseases of the CNS in which a viral etiology is suspected, among which is multiple sclerosis.

Unconventional or True Slow Viral Infections

Slow viral infections were first named and described in Iceland. In a series of papers in 1954, Sigurdsson *et al.* (1957) discussed three chronic diseases of sheep: Maedi, a slow, progressive pneumonia; Rida, a chronic encephalitis either closely related or identical to scrapie; and Johne's disease, a paratuberculosis. Later on, visna, a progressive, demyelinating, and transmissible viral infection of sheep, was added to the list (Sigurdsson *et al.*, 1957). Scrapie and its transmissibility had already been described by Cuille as early as 1936 (Cuille, 1938).

The criteria used by Sigurdsson for slow infections were: (1) a very long initial period of latency lasting from several months to several years; (2) a rather regular protracted course after clinical signs have appeared, usually ending in serious disease or death; and (3) limitation of the infection to a single host species, and anatomical lesions in only a single organ or tissue system (though this criterion was later modified to consider a wider host susceptibility). The visna–maedi complex shares characteristics with some retroviruses, such as the human immunodeficiency virus (HIV). Visna has been called a slow virus infection because of the long incubation period, but it does not belong to the unconventional group. On the other hand, scrapie, so named because itching of the skin lesions makes the sheep scrape themselves against objects, is caused by the prototype of a group of viruses called unconventional or true slow viruses. It is noninflammatory in nature and produces no detectable immune response. Also, nucleic acid is not present in the agent.

The unconventional group includes scrapie, transmissible mink encephalopathy, and three human diseases, kuru, Creutzfeldt–Jakob disease (CJD), and Gerstmann-Straüssler-Schenker syndrome (GSS). They are referred to as the spongioform encephalitides because of the spongy appearance of the pathological changes found in the brain. The features of the agents and of the host response are shown in Table 4.1. The extraordinarily high resistance of the viruses to heat, ultraviolet light, and various chemicals, such as formalin, and the long incubation period in both animals and humans are key features, in addition to those already mentioned. There is some question about whether they should be called viruses, because they do not have nucleic acid (DNA, RNA), which characterizes all conventional viruses. Prusinger (1982) and Prusinger *et al.* (1983) claim to have identified a small, infectious protein and refer to the infectious agent as prions. This work initially needed further confirmation because the components identified might have been products of the host tissue rather than the agent itself. Currently, the results are generally accepted. From the standpoint of establishing causation, these unconventional agents pose special problems because the agent cannot be isolated and grown in culture and the infection does not result in a detectable immune response. This means that none of the criteria thus far described is applicable to the group. Before proceeding with the current criteria of causation, a description of the human diseases may be of interest.

Epidemiologically, kuru is a fascinating disease. It was first described in the medical literature by Gajdusek and Zigas (1957). They observed it in the Fore tribe, a group of primitive people living in the highlands of Papua, New Guinea, where it remains geographically restricted. Clinically, kuru is a progressive and fatal neurological disease of about 24 months' average duration.

The disease was recognized in the first or second decade of the 20th century

Table 4.1

Subacute Spongioform Virus Encephalopathies (Unconventional Viruses) of Humans and Animals and Their Characteristics[a]

Viruses	
Of humans:	Kuru (limited to New Guinea)
	Creutzfeldt–Jakob disease (familial and sporadic)
	Gerstmann–Straussler disease (familial and sporadic)
Of animals	Scrapie of sheep and goats
	Transmissible mink encephalopathy
	Chronic wasting disease of mule deer and captive elk
	Bovine spongioform encephalopathy
Characteristics:	Long incubation period
	Contain no DNA or RNA, but contain "prions"
	Not visualizable under the electron microscope
	Induce no detectable antibody response
	Multiply to high titers in appropriate tissues
	Highly resistant to heat, ultraviolet light, many chemicals
	Amyloid fibrils seen in infected brain resembling aggregated scrapie-associated protein ("prion")

[a] Derived in part from Gibbs (1989).

and rates slowly increased until they reached epidemic proportions during the 1950s (Gajdusek, 1973). In 1956, intensive studies were begun and the possibility of a simple genetic hypothesis and of an infectious origin was investigated, with no conclusive results. We owe much of our knowledge of the epidemiology and etiology of kuru to the work of Carleton Gajdusek (Figure 4.1) and his associates at the National Institutes of Health. A case registry was established. The disease was found to be confined to members of about 160 villages, with a total population of 35,000, among whom over 2500 cases have been identified since 1956, primarily in the Fore linguistic group. At one point, up to 200 deaths from kuru occurred yearly. Among preadolescents the sex ratio was about equal, but in adults there was a 3:1 female predominance, which has been dropping toward 1:1 in the last decade.

The most striking aspects of the disease are the method of transmission and the long incubation period. Ritual cannibalism was introduced in about 1920, and consumption of a dead kinsman, particularly his brain, as an act of mourning appeared to be the main method of transmission. Women prepared the body bare-handed and squeezed brain tissue in bamboo cylinders, in which it was steamed. The virus is highly resistant to heat, and the low boiling temperature, 90–95 °C, in the mountainous area may have failed to inactivate it. Adult men rarely participated in this ceremony and seldom ate the flesh of the kuru victims; the

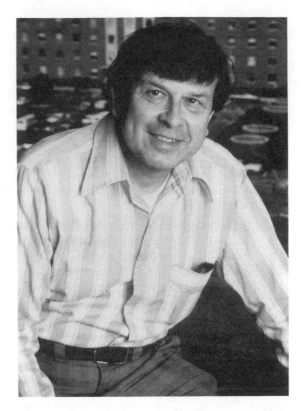

Figure 4.1. Dr. Carleton Gajdusek, 1923– , Chief, Laboratory of Central Nervous System Studies, National Institute of Neurological and Communicative Disorders and Stroke, National Institutes of Health.

women and children were primarily at risk. Both ingestion of the contaminated brain tissue and absorption through abrasions in the skin were possible mechanisms of transmission of the agent. The gradual decline in the incidence of the disease since cannibalism was discontinued from 1957 to 1962, and the observation that no child under 10 years old has developed kuru since 1967 support this idea of the means of transmission. Recent epidemiological studies of three funeral feasts and on follow-up of those who attended them, undertaken by Klitzman, as part of his Yale medical thesis and published in conjunction with Gajdusek and Alpers (Klitzman *et al.*, 1984), have indicated several important points: (1) the incubation period can range from 6 to 28 years or more (earlier evidence had suggested a period as short as 3 years), can be identical in two or more individuals infected simultaneously, and is not determined by the patient's age at the time of exposure; (2) kuru is transmitted at the time of cannibalistic mourning; (3) the attack rate among those participating in the feasts may exceed 77%. The establishment of an infectious etiology of the disease was successful in 1966 when Gajdusek and his associates transmitted the disease to chimpanzees, based on the earlier suggestion of Hadlow (1959) that there were neuropathological similarities between scrapie and kuru. The disease developed 20 months after the intracerebral inoculation of human brain tissue from kuru patients, thus providing experimental evidence of a long incubation period. Gajdusek was awarded the Nobel Prize for his work with kuru. The disease, as well as Creutzfeldt–Jakob and scrapie, was later transmitted experimentally by the oral route to nonhuman primates, amplifying the evidence for cannibalism as the route of transmission (Gibbs *et al.*, 1980).

Creutzfeldt–Jakob disease (CJD), another chronic neurological disease caused by a slow virus, was described in the early 1920s, is worldwide in distribution, and has an incidence of about one per million (Gibbs, 1989). The agent, itself, is indistinguishable from that of kuru by current virological methods. About 90% of cases occur in adults aged 40–69 years with about an equal sex distribution. The disease was transmitted, through infected brain tissue, to chimpanzees by Gibbs (Figure 4.2) and associates (1968), and later to smaller experimental animals by Manuelides and colleagues (Manuelides *et al.*, 1976a, 1977, 1978). While the natural route of transmission in humans is unknown, transmission has been shown to occur via infected cornea (Manuelides *et al.*, 1977) and by stereotactic electroencephalographic (EEG) electrodes that had

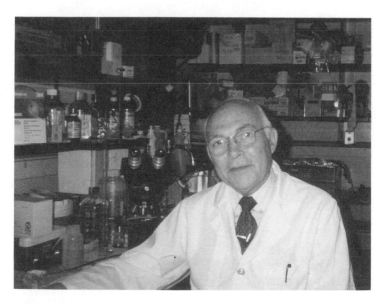

Figure 4.2. Dr. Clarence J. Gibbs, Jr., 1924– , Laboratory of Central Nervous System Studies, National Institute of Neurological and Communicative Disorders and Stroke, National Institutes of Health.

been previously used on a CJD patient (Bernouilli *et al.*, 1979). A neurosurgeon apparently contracted the disease after he stabbed himself with a lancet while operating on a CJD patient. More recently, two types of infection have occurred from the use of cadaver materials. One involved the use of human dura mater from a German tissue bank on persons with breaks in their dura mater needing repair (Centers for Disease Control, 1987, 1989). The other resulted from the use of growth hormone in seven children, using material derived from the pituitary gland of cadavers (Centers for Disease Control, 1985). Obviously, any cadaver tissues derived from patients with fatal chronic neurological diseases should not be used in the future, even though the estimated incidence of CJD is about one in a million. If used in a pool of materials, such as growth hormones, it might contaminate large lots and infect many persons. In addition to this, the possibility that inapparent carriers of such viruses exist has not yet been completely excluded.

The inability to isolate the agents of kuru and CJD in tissue culture or to demonstrate an immunological response to them led to the proposal of a new set of guidelines by Johnson (Figure 4.4) and Gibbs (1974) for relating slow viral infections to chronic neurological disease, as shown in Table 4.2. The consistent, serial experimental reproduction of the disease in experimental animals in more than one laboratory is the key recommendation. The demonstration of the agent

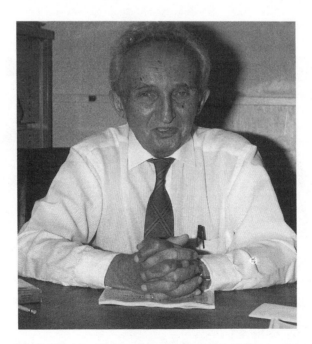

Figure 4.3. Dr. Elias E. Manuelides, 1918–1992, Professor of Neuropathology, emeritus, Yale University School of Medicine.

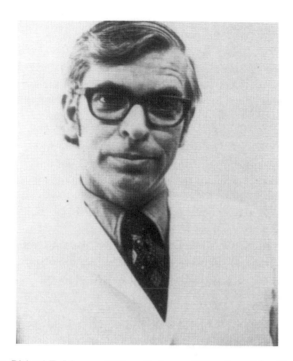

Figure 4.4. Dr. Richard T. Johnson, 1931– , Professor of Neurology, Johns Hopkins University School of Medicine.

itself in diseased tissues through the electron microscope, through immunofluorescence techniques, or even using current molecular biological methods is not yet possible for the agents of kuru or CJD. The third criterion, that tests of normal tissues or tissues from patients with other diseases should be carried out to establish that the agent is not a ubiquitous one, does not eliminate the possibility that latent, asymptomatic infections of the CNS may occur, even with the slow viruses. The isolation of the CJD agent by Manuelides in guinea pigs that had been inoculated with biopsy material from the brain of a patient who subsequently recovered indicates that recovery may occur (Manuelides *et al.*, 1978). Indeed, several viral agents, such as herpes simplex virus or varicella-zoster virus, may lie latent in the brain of normal or diseased persons. When brain tissue from a patient with some other chronic neurological disease is inoculated into an experimental animal, then these viruses might produce some other disease without being the cause of the disease under study. This problem of the carrier state was one of the limitations to the second of Koch's original postulates, that "the parasite should occur in no other disease as a fortuitous and nonpathogenic parasite." One can expect that advances in molecular virology will eventually provide modifications to Johnson's and Gibbs's guidelines and will eliminate some of these questions. Even with the limited evidence now

Table 4.2
**Johnson's and Gibbs's Criteria for Relating Slow Viral Infections and Chronic
Neurological Disease**[a]

---

1. There should be consistency in the transmission of the disease to experimental animals or some consistency in the recovery of the virus in cell cultures, and this transmission or recovery should be confirmed by more than one laboratory.
2. Either serial transmission of the clinicopathological process should be accomplished using filtered material and serial dilutions to establish replication of the agent, or the recoverable agent should be demonstrated with consistency in the diseased tissue by electron microscopic, immunofluorescent, or other methods, and should be demonstrated in the appropriate cells to explain the lesions.
3. Parallel studies of normal tissues or tissues of patients with other diseases should be carried out to establish that the agent is not a ubiquitous agent or a contaminant.

---

[a]From Johnson and Gibbs (1974)

available, there are few who doubt that these unconventional slow viruses are the cause of kuru and CJD and are probably infectious agents called prions (Prusinger, 1992).

Chronic CNS Diseases Due to Conventional Viruses

There are several viruses or groups of viruses of the conventional type containing nucleic acids, i.e., DNA or RNA, that produce an immune response, albeit often an abnormal one, and that can result in chronic infections of the CNS. This complication is a rare event. Viruses capable of producing persistent neural infections include herpesviruses, adenoviruses, papovaviruses, rhabdoviruses, retroviruses, coronaviruses, arenaviruses, togaviruses, and picornaviruses (Johnson, 1982). The mechanism by which persistence occurs and the mechanisms involved in the destruction of myelin in the nervous system vary with different viruses. Viral infections can cause demyelination without involving the immune system, or via virus-induced immune response, or by nonspecific mechanisms, or possibly by disruption of immune regulation. Several of these viruses are capable of synthesis of antibodies in the CNS (Salmi *et al.*, 1983a,b). The causal evidence supporting a relationship between two of these viruses and the chronic nervous-system diseases with which they are associated will be discussed below.

Subacute Sclerosing Pan Encephalitis (SSPE)

This is a chronic and progressive neurological disease with onset in children, often as a reading or behavioral problem, and then leading to seizures and death. It is associated with a measleslike virus. Epidemiologically, the disease is worldwide but rare, with an incidence ranging from 0.12 to 1.4 per million; about 40 new cases are reported yearly in the United States (Gibbs, 1989). Males outnumber females about 3:1. The most striking finding is a history of measles infection early in life: in some studies, over half of the cases have such a history in the first 2 years of life. The evidence of a causal relationship includes: (1) the presence of defective measles antigen in the brains of SSPE patients, as demonstrated by the electron microscope or immunofluorescent antibody techniques, and the isolation of a measleslike virus by cocultivation from the brain; (2) the presence of high levels of measles antibody in the serum and significant titers of both IgG and IgM antibody in the cerebrospinal fluid (CSF) of most patients, indicating antibody synthesis within the CNS; and (3) the reproduction of some of the features of the disease in two experimental animal models using a hamster-adapted measles virus. This evidence establishes a firm causal link between measleslike viruses and SSPE, but one probably dependent on a defective virus and/or a defect in the immune system of the host. In addition, other viruses like rubella and Epstein–Barr virus may rarely result in the same clinical syndrome.

Progressive Multifocal Leukoencephalopathy (PML)

PML is also a rare, demyelinating disease of the CNS, with death occurring some 2–4 months after the onset of symptoms (Zu Rhein, 1982). Some 200–250 cases have been reported in the world literature since its first description by Zu Rhein (Figure 4.5) and Chow (1965), when viral particles resembling papovavirus were found in the brains of Hodgkin's disease patients dying of a progressive neurological disease. It occurs mostly in adults age 50–70, but there have been a couple of cases in children. Recently, it has occurred in adults with AIDS, appearing in from 3.8% (Krupp et al., 1985) to 6.7% (Lang et al., 1989) of AIDS cases. Geographically, the cases have been reported from developed countries: the United States, Canada, European countries, Australia, and Japan (Gibbs, 1989). Most cases have occurred in hypergic individuals as a late complication of a preexisting, generalized systemic disease; over half of the cases have been in patients with lymphoproliferative or myeloproliferative diseases, such as Hodgkin's disease and chronic lymphatic leukemia. The possible viral etiology of the disease was first reported by Zu Rhein and Chow (1965) when papovalike particles were found by electron microscopy in the brains of PML

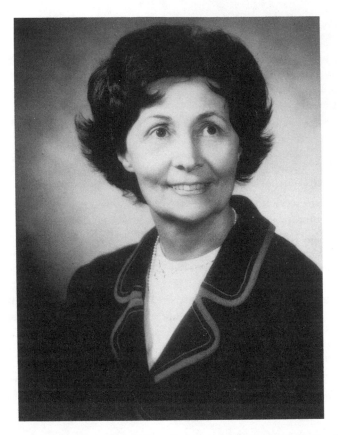

Figure 4.5. Dr. Gabriele Zu Rhein, 1920– , Professor of Pathology, University of Wisconsin School of Medicine.

patients. The virus was isolated by Padgett and associates in 1971 in human fetal brain cells, and antibody to the agent was found to be present in over 65% of healthy children by age 14 in Wisconsin (Padgett and Walker, 1973). The viral strain was designated as JC for the patient from whom it was isolated. It is a polyomavirus in the papova family of viruses, whose other member is termed papillomavirus (which includes the wart virus and some strains associated with cervical cancer). No clinical disease has been identified in association with the primary infection with the JL strain. This strain has been found most commonly in the brains of PML patients, although another strain of the polyomavirus, SV-40 or simian virus 40, was initially implicated in a few cases, but this evidence is now questioned (Stoner, 1991).

The evidence relating the agent to the disease includes (1) the constant demonstration of the virus in the brains of PML patients by electron microscopy, immunofluorescence, or viral isolation, and (2) the presence of antibody to the agent, often in high titer, in the serum of patients. The missing evidence is that infection with the virus and the appearance of antibody have not been shown to precede the onset of the disease. A question is thus raised whether the disease might represent a primary infection in an immunocompromised host, a reactivated and causally related viral infection occurring years after the primary infection (which seems most likely in view of the high frequency of childhood infection), or simply a reactivated infection unrelated causally to the disease. Epidemiologically, demonstration of the more frequent occurrence of the disease in persons with papovavirus antibody than in those without would be desirable. The rarity of the disease, however, precludes the possibility of showing any of these time relationships in prospective studies. Additionally, the disease has not been reproduced experimentally in animals, although inoculation of the virus intracerebrally into hamsters and monkeys has resulted in brain tumors (Walker *et al.*, 1973; London *et al.*, 1978). Thus, both PML and SSPE probably represent very rare manifestations of the reactivation of prior infection by common and ubiquitous viruses in persons with a natural or drug-induced immunodeficiency, but the factors precipitating the disease in so few persons among those infected with the virus remain unknown, except the increasing frequency of PML in patients with AIDS (Krupp *et al.*, 1985; Lang *et al.*, 1989). An increasing number of cases of progressive multifocal leukoencephalopathy (PML) in patients with HIV infection or AIDS is due in part to the longer life expectancy provided by AZT therapy. In 1987, sixteen new cases of PML were reported in HIV-infected persons, and an additional twelve reviewed from the literature (Berger *et al.*, 1987). The number has grown since then. In some cases, PML is the initial clinical manifestation of AIDS. The virus can now be identified in brain tissue using the polymerase chain reaction (PCR) (Telenti *et al.*, 1990), and newer radiological techniques, such as magnetic resonance imaging, are permitting clinical diagnosis.

New Challenges

The discovery that certain chronic diseases of the CNS are due to viruses has led to the possibility that other diseases, such as multiple sclerosis, Alzheimer's disease, and amyotrophic lateral sclerosis (Gehrig's disease) might have a similar etiology. The most extensive work in this area has been done on multiple sclerosis (MS), and the most false etiological leads have been encountered with this disease, which is the most common and best known of the demyelinating afflictions of the human CNS. It occurs worldwide but with much higher incidence in colder climates. The onset of the disease is usually after age 15 with a peak about age 30. Persons born in the higher-risk, colder areas who migrate to a low-risk, warmer area after the age of 15 carry with them the high risk of their native area, although the disease may not develop until 20 years later; if migration occurs before the age of 15, the risk of MS is that of the low-risk area. This suggests an early environmental factor. Genetic factors may also be important because the disease is 15–20 times more common in first-degree relatives of MS patients than in unrelated persons. The evidence suggesting that MS may have an infectious disease etiology includes the different geographic distribution, familial aggregation, clustering of cases such as in the Shetland and Orkney islands (where there are 128 cases per 100,000 population), and the migrant studies already mentioned. These epidemiological features might also be associated with an environmental or genetic hypothesis with or without a viral connection. Some of the candidate infectious agents and their causal evidence will be discussed. The agents include measles virus (Norrby and Vankid, 1974; Norrby, 1978), distemper virus (Cook and Dowling, 1980), and MS-associated agent (MSSA) (Koldovsky et al., 1975; Henle et al., 1975). Brown and Gadjusek (1974) and Nathanson and Miller (1978) were unable to confirm the findings for MSSA, finally leading to a withdrawal of the claim by the original authors (Carp et al., 1977). Then there is the agent isolated by Mitchell et al. (1978) which was denied by Micheletti et al. (1979), the virus isolated by Melnick (1982) and Melnick et al. (1982), and more recently the human T-cell leukemia viruses (Koprowski et al., 1985).

Before proceeding further in this discussion, some of the features of the viruses and of antibody in relation to the pathogenesis of the disease deserve comment. Viruses could produce demyelinating injury to the nervous system in three ways, as pointed out by Waksman (1983) and Waksman et al. (1984): (1) a virus could directly infect and damage oligodendrocytes and produce myelin breakdown and perhaps some degree of inflammation; (2) an immunological response to the persistent viral antigens in the white matter of the brain can result in an inflammatory response and some degree of secondary demyelination; (3) an autoimmune response might occur from the viral infection, either as a result of cross-reactivity to some component of the oligodendrocyte or the myelin, or as a consequence of tissue damage and the release of autoantigen at the time of the initial infection. A population of helper T cells specific for the virus might provide a strong nonspecific adjuvant effect and promote the immune response against the autoantigen. It should be noted that the first of these mechanisms would require a specific etiological agent or agents with special characteristics. The second and third might occur with many viruses that could persist, immunize, and lead to immunization and/or autoimmunization. The presence of antibody to the suspected viral agent, even in high titer, and even when antibody is produced in the CNS can be a nonspecific phenomenon. This latter point deserves emphasis because the relationship to some of the candidate viruses has been based on intrathecal production of specific antibody, sometimes of the IgM type. While the CNS does not normally make antibody, it can do so in acute infections of the CNS and in demyelinating diseases: at least 16 viruses have been shown to do this in MS and sometimes several antibodies are produced simultaneously (Salmi *et al.,* 1983a,b). Thus, the finding of antibody to a particular virus in the CNS lacks the specificity required for a strong causal relationship.

Let us now briefly review the strength of the association with some of the candidate viruses. Measles virus is perhaps the best documented. In some 25 studies of measles antibody titers in the sera of MS patients as compared to controls, modest but often significantly high titers have been found in most of the investigations. Measles antibody of the IgG type, but not the IgM type, has been found in the CSF of patients, but not in that of controls (Norrby and Vankid, 1974). Antibodies to the nucleoprotein components of the measles virus have been elevated more consistently and to higher titer than antibodies to the viral envelope. However, as noted above, other viral antibodies may also be present in the CSF of MS patients, of which rubella virus, vaccinia virus, and the herpesviruses have been the most common. The antibody findings for measles virus in MS are not nearly so impressive and specific as in SSPE, discussed previously in this chapter. While measles virus has been isolated from a case of postmeasles encephalitis, a common complication of the disease, it has not been isolated from, or demonstrated in, the brain of MS patients, in contrast to SSPE patients. A close relative of measles virus, distemper virus, has also been incriminated in an interesting epidemiological setting in the Faroe Islands. Antibody to this virus is very difficult to distinguish from that of measles virus, and there is no direct evidence that humans are naturally infected by distemper virus, although the reverse might be true in dogs (i.e., there may be evidence of measles virus infection in dogs).

Measles has been long recognized in the Faroe Islands since Panum described the first epidemic of the disease in a classic paper in 1846 (Panum, 1948). Distemper virus was apparently introduced in 1940 during the British occupation of the islands. MS had been absent from native Faroe Islanders but appeared in three epidemic waves of decreasing size beginning in 1943, three years after the start of the British occupation of the islands in 1940 during which they were accompanied by their dogs. In very careful epidemiological studies of this outbreak by Kurtzke (Kurtzke, 1980, 1987; Kurtzke and Hyllested, 1979, 1985, 1987; Kurtzke and Priester, 1979), he and his colleagues found 25 cases after 1943 in Faroe Islanders who had not been off the island and 7 cases in persons off the island less than 2 years. They feel that the first wave was due to an asymptomatic agent introduced by the British and that later waves were the result of transmission among the Faroe Islanders. They postulate that MS is due to a single infectious agent, transmissible at most from age 13 to 26, that is asymptomatic and leads in rare instances to neurological involvement (Kurtzke, 1987). In contrast to Cook and Dowling (1980), they do not believe this agent to be distemper virus because they have found no evidence of a relationship in epidemiological studies carried out in the United States, and others have failed to find distemper-specific antibody in MS cases. The issue remains controversial (Stephenson *et al.,* 1991).

A third candidate cause of MS, about which there was much early excitement, was MSSA, and the evidence was both virological and immunological (Koldovsky *et al.,* 1975; Henle *et al.,* 1975). A transitory depression of the leukocyte count of mice, rats, hamsters, and guinea pigs was regularly induced on inoculation of brain tissue suspension from eight cases of MS, and antibody to the filterable agent was also found frequently in high titer in the serum of these patients. It could be serially transmitted from animal to animal. No agent was isolated from control materials. Neutralizing activity present in the immunoglobulin fraction was found in sera from 20 of 22 MS patients as well as in their CSF. It was also found in sera from relatives of MS patients, as well as their nursing personnel, but very rarely in sera from patients with other diseases or from healthy American controls. Sera from over half of East African donors showed neutralizing activity, suggesting that the agent might be more common in developing countries. However, other investigators could not confirm these results (Brown and Gajdusek, 1974), and when coded specimens were submitted to the original workers, they were unable to distinguish between material from MS patients and that of controls (Nathanson and Miller, 1978). A retraction from the original authors resulted (Carp *et al.,* 1977). Newer candidate agents have been reported in a preliminary fashion by Mitchell *et al.* (1978) but then quickly denied (Mitchell *et al.,* 1979). Another virus has been apparently isolated by Melnick *et al.* (1982), but the results must be confirmed by others.

Perhaps the most interesting new possible causes are the human T-cell leukemia retroviruses (HTLV). Recent evidence has demonstrated the presence of antibodies reactive with HTLV antigens in the CSF of MS patients from Sweden, in concentrations significantly higher than in other neurological diseases or healthy controls, as well as higher titers of antibodies to the p24 and disrupted HTLV antigens than in the other groups (Koprowski *et al.,* 1985). They also found that 10 of 17 sera from MS patients in Key West, Florida, reacted at one time or another with an HTLV antigen, as compared with only 2 of 17 sera from close contacts of the patients, one of whom was a homosexual with HTLV-III antibody, and with none of 17 sera from hospital staff workers from the same area. The antibodies found varied in their occurrence in both sera and CSF, were not present in all patients' sera, and reacted differently with various HTLV antigens, suggesting that it was different from HTLV-I, -II, or -III. No virus has thus far been isolated. In other studies, however, the human immunodeficiency virus (HIV) has been identified in both acute and chronic neurological diseases with or without the usual manifestations of AIDS; thus, cells of the nervous system as well as the T4 lymphocyte may be targets for the virus. A new era of agents responsible for CNS diseases has therefore opened with the discovery of the relation of human retroviruses to the brain. At present, much more work and confirmatory studies need to be done in different laboratories to confirm the importance of this group of persistent viruses.

In summary, the viral etiology of MS has not been established by any of the criteria so far discussed, and the strength of the association with any of the candidate agents is currently too weak to point firmly to a virus as *the* cause of MS. Even if a virus causes MS, it is not clear if it is a single agent, as suggested by Kurtzke and Hyllested (1987), or any one of several that are persistent and can invoke an autoimmune response against elements of the CNS, as Waksman (1981, 1983) and Reynolds (1984) suggest. I hold to the latter hypothesis and believe the cause may vary in different geographic locations and in different epidemiological settings. However, if there were a single cause, it would have the advantage that a vaccine might be developed against it that might prevent MS.

Summary

The information presented in this chapter provides firm evidence that kuru and CJD cause the spongioform encephalitides with which they are associated, mainly based on experimental reproduction of these fatal neurological diseases in laboratory animals. There is also strong virological and epidemiological evidence that SSPE can result from measles virus or its variant, when infection occurs very early in life, although other viruses like Epstein–Barr or rubella, on rare occasions, are also associated with this syndrome. Similarly, PML is due to a common papovavirus (the JC strain) in which reactivation occurs in the presence of immunodeficiency. To date, virus or viruses have been linked to MS in association with an aberrant immune response, but the specific agents that cause this have not been conclusively identified, and investigation of this etiology has proven to be a hazard to many fine investigators.

A new hypothesis has tried to bring together some common pathogenetic events for these chronic neurological syndromes caused by slow viruses (Gibbs, 1989). It is based on the pathological changes seen in neurofibrillary tangles (NFT) and amyloid plaques, which are similar to those seen in the aging brain. The NFT are seen in infections of the brain in SSPE and in chronic rubella infections, and the amyloid plaques have been observed with certain strains of scrapie, kuru, and CJD in the appropriate natural hosts. But similar lesions have also been found in patients suffering from aluminum intoxication, and in dialysis dementia. It is thus possible that several viruses, toxic or genetic determinants, or perhaps even trauma may lead to the lesions with NFT and amyloid plaques. The underlying mechanism is postulated to be interference with axonal transport of neurofilaments. Modern developments in molecular virology and protein chemistry may shed light on the hypothesis that self-replicating proteins resembling "viruses" can result in the autocatalytic patterned degeneration of host precursor proteins to amyloid (Gibbs, 1989). A strong case has been presented that infectious proteins called "prions" are a major cause of these "slow viral infections" (Prusinger, 1992) and are related to amyloid materials (Prusinger *et al.*, 1983). Amyloid derivatives might thus become transformed into self-replicating agents under certain provoking determinants. Such new evidence will pose new challenges in establishing the proof of causation and the risk factors involved in these fascinating chronic neurological syndromes.

References

Astrom KE, Mancell EL, Richardson EP Jr: Progressive focal leukoencephalopathy. *Brain* **81**:93–111, 1954.

Bernouilli C, Sigfried J, Baumgarten C, *et al:* Danger of accidental person-to-person transmission of Creutzfeldt–Jakob disease by surgery. *Lancet* **1**:478–479, 1979.

Brown P, Gajdusek DC: No mouse PMN leukocyte depression after inoculation with brain tissue from multiple sclerosis or spongioform encephalopathy. *Nature* **247**:217–218, 1974.

Brown P, Tsai T, Gajdusek DC: Seroepidemiology of human papovavirus. Discovery of virgin populations and some unusual patterns of antibody prevalence among remote people of the world. *Am J Epidemiol* **102**:331–340, 1975.

Carp RE, Licuse PC, Merz PA, *et al:* Letter to editor. Multiple sclerosis-associated agent. *Lancet* **2**:814, 1977.

Centers for Disease Control: Fatal degenerative neurological disease in patients who received pituitary-derived growth hormone. *MMWR* **34**:359–360, 365–366, 1985.

Centers for Disease Control: Rapidly progressive dementia in a patient who received a cadaveric dura mater graft. *MMWR* **36**:49–50, 55, 1987.

Centers for Disease Control: Update: Creutzfeldt–Jakob disease in a second patient who received cadaveric dura mater graft. *MMWR* **38**:37–38, 43, 1989.

Cook SD, Dowling PD: Multiple sclerosis and viruses: An overview. *Neurology* **30**:80–91, 1980.

Cuille J, and Chello PL: Las "tremblante" de mouton est bien inoculable. *Comptes rendus des seances de l'Academie des Sci Paris* **206**:78–79, 1938.

Gajdusek C, Zigas V: Degenerative disease of the central nervous system in New Guinea. The endemic occurrence of "kuru" in the native population. *N Engl J Med* **257**:974, 1957.

Gajdusek DC: Kuru and Creutzfeldt–Jakob disease. *Ann Clin Res* **5**:254, 1973.

Gajdusek DC: Slow infections with unconventional viruses. *Harvey Lect* **72**:283–353, 1978.

Gajdusek DC, Gibbs CJ Jr: Subacute and chronic diseases caused by atypical infection with unconventional viruses in aberrant hosts, in Pollard M (ed): *Persistent Virus Infections, Perspectives in Virology* vol 8. New York, Academic Press, 1973, pp 279–301.

Gajdusek DC, Gibbs CJ Jr, Alpers M: Experimental transmission of a kuru-like syndrome to chimpanzees. *Nature* **209**:794–796, 1966.

Gibbs CJ Jr: Chronic neurological diseases. Subacute sclerosing panencephalitis, progressive multifocal leukoencephalopathy, kuru, Creutzfeldt–Jakob disease, in Evans AS (ed): *Viral Infections of Humans: Epidemiology and Control*, 3rd ed. New York, Plenum Press, 1989, pp 781–806.

Gibbs CJ Jr, Gajdusek DC, Asher DM, *et al:* Creutzfeldt–Jakob disease (spongioform encephalopathy): Transmission to the chimpanzee. *Science* **161:**388–389, 1968.

Gibbs CJ Jr, Amyx WL, Bacote A, *et al:* Oral transmission of kuru, Creutzfeldt–Jakob disease, and scrapie to non-human primates. *J Infect Dis* **142:**205–208, 1980.

Hadlow WJ: Scrapie and kuru. *Lancet* **2:**289–290, 1959.

Henle G, Henle W, Koldovsky P, *et al:* Multiple sclerosis-associated agent: Neutralization of the agent by human sera. *Infect Immun* **12:**1367–1374, 1975.

Johnson RT: *Viral Infections of the Nervous System.* New York, Raven Press, 1982.

Johnson R, Gibbs CJ Jr: Editorial. Koch's postulates and slow infections of the nervous system. *Arch Neurol* **30:**36–38, 1974.

Klitzman RL, Alpers MP, Gajdusek DC: The natural incubation period of kuru and the episodes of transmission in three clusters of patients. *Neuroepidemiology* **3:**3–20, 1984.

Koldovsky U, Koldovsky P, Henle G, *et al:* Studies on a multiple sclerosis-associated agent— Transmission to animals and some properties of the agent. *Infect Immun* **12:**1355–1366, 1975.

Koprowski H, DeFreiltas EC, Harper ME, *et al:* Multiple sclerosis and human T-cell lymphotropic retrovirus. *Nature* **318:**154–160, 1985.

Krupp LB, Lipton RB, Swerlow ML, *et al:* Progressive multifocal leukoencephalopathy: Clinical and radiologic features. *Ann Neurol* **17:**244–349, 1985.

Kurtzke JF: Epidemiologic contributions to multiple sclerosis. An overview. *Neurology* **30:**61–79, 1980.

Kurtzke JF: Multiple sclerosis in the Faroe Islands. III. An alternative assessment of the three epidemics. *Act Neurol Scand* **76:**317–319, 1987.

Kurtzke JF, Hyllested K: Multiple sclerosis in the Faroe Islands: I. Clinical and epidemiological features. *Ann Neurol* **5:**6–21, 1979.

Kurtzke JF, Hyllested K: Multiple sclerosis in the Faroe Islands: II. Clinical update, transmission, and the nature of MS. *Neurology* **35:**672–676, 1985.

Kurtzke JF, Hyllested K: MS epidemiology in the Faroe Islands. *Rev Neurol* **57:**77–87, 1987.

Kurtzke JF, Priester WA: Dogs, distemper, and multiple sclerosis in the United States. *Acta Neurol Scand* **60:**313–319, 1979.

Lang W, Miklossy J, Deranz JP, *et al:* Neuropathology of the acquired immunodeficiency syndrome (AIDS). Report of 135 consecutive autopsy cases from Switzerland. *Acta Neuropath* **77:**379–380, 1989.

London WT, Houff SA, Madden DL, *et al:* Brain tumors in owl monkeys with polyoma virus (JE virus). *Science* **201:**1246–1249, 1978.

Manuelides EE, Gorgacz EJ, Manuelides L: Interspecies transmission of Creutzfeldt–Jakob disease to the Syrian hamster with reference to clinical syndromes and strains of agent. *Proc Natl Acad Sci USA* **75:**3432–3436, 1976a.

Manuelides EE, Kim J, Angelo JN, *et al:* Serial propagation of Creutzfeldt–Jakob disease in guinea pigs. *Proc Natl Acad Sci USA* **73:**223–227, 1976b.

Manuelides EE, Angelo JN, Gorgacz EJ, *et al:* Experimental Creutzfeldt–Jakob disease transmitted via the eye with infected cornea. *N Engl J Med* **296:**1334–1336, 1977.

Manuelides EE, Manuelides L, Pincus JH, *et al:* Transmission from man to the hamster of Creutzfeldt–Jakob disease with clinical recovery. *Lancet* **2:**40–42, 1978.

Melnick JL: Has the virus of multiple sclerosis been isolated? *Yale J Biol Med* **55:**251–257, 1982.

Melnick JL, Seide EL, Inoue YK, *et al:* Isolation of virus from spinal fluid of three patients with multiple sclerosis and one with amyotropic lateral sclerosis. *Lancet* **1:**30–33, 1982.

Micheletti R, Lange LS, Jakob JP, *et al:* Failure to isolate a transmissible agent from the bone marrow of patients with multiple sclerosis. *Lancet* **2:**415–416, 1979.

Mitchell DN, Porterfield JS, Micheletti R, *et al:* Isolation of an infectious agent from bone marrow of patients with multiple sclerosis. *Lancet* **2:**387–391, 1978.

Mitchell DN, Goswami KK, Taylor P, *et al*: Failure to isolate a transmissible agent from the bone marrow of patients with multiple sclerosis. *Lancet* **2:**415–416, 1979.

Nathanson N, Miller A: Epidemiology of multiple sclerosis. Critique of the evidence for a viral etiology. *Am J Epidemiol* **107:**451–461, 1978.

Norrby E: Viral antibodies in multiple sclerosis. *Prog Med Virol* **24:**1–39, 1978.

Norrby E, Vankid B: Measles and multiple sclerosis. *Proc R Soc Med* **67:**1129–1132, 1974.

Padgett BL, Walker DL: Prevalence of antibodies in human sera against JC virus, an isolate from a case of progressive multifocal leukoencephalopathy. *J Infect Dis* **127:**467–470, 1973.

Padgett BL, Zu Rhein GM, Walker DL, *et al:* Cultivation of papova-like virus from human brain with progressive multifocal leukencephalopathy. *Lancet* **1:**1257–1260, 1971.

Panum PL: *Observations Made during the Epidemic of Measles in the Faroe Islands in the Year 1846.* New York, American Public Health Association, 1948.

Prusinger SB: Novel proteinaceous infectious particles cause scrapie. *Science* **216:**136–144, 1982.

Prusinger SB, McKinley MP, Bowman KA, *et al:* Scrapie prions aggregate to form amyloid-like birefrigent rods. *Cell* **35:**349–358, 1983.

Prusinger SB: Molecular biology and genetics of neurodegenerative diseases caused by prions. *Adv Virus Res* **41:**241–380, 1992.

Salmi A, Arnadottir T, Reulnanen *et al:* The significance of antibody synthesis in the central nervous system of multiple sclerosis patients, in Mims CA, Cruzner ML, Kelly RE (eds): *Viruses and Demyelinating Diseases.* New York, Academic Press, 1983a, pp 141–154.

Salmi A, Reunanen M, Leonen J, *et al:* Intrathecal antibody synthesis to virus antigens in multiple sclerosis. *Clin Exp Immunol* **52:**239–241, 1983b.

Sigurdsson B: Observation on three slow infections of sheep. *Br Med J* **110:**255, 307, 341, 1954.

Sigurdsson B, Palsson PA, Grimsson H: Visna, a demyelinating transmissible disease of sheep. *J Neuropathol Exp Neurol* **15:**389–403, 1957.

Stephenson JR, ter Meulen V, Kiessling W: Search for canine distemper virus antibodies in multiple sclerosis. A detailed virological evaluation. *Lancet* **2:**772–775, 1980.

Stoner GL: Implications of progressive multifocal leukoencephalopathy and JC virus for the etiology of MS. *Acta Neurol Scand* **83:**20–33, 1991.

Telente A, *et al*: Detection of JC virus by polymerase chain reaction in cerebrospinal fluid from two patients with progressive multifocal leukoencephalopathy. *Eur J Clin Microbiol Infect Dis* **11:**253–254, 1992.

Waksman BH: Current trends in multiple sclerosis research. *Immunol Today* 87–93, 1981.

Waksman BH: Viruses and immune events in the pathogenesis of multiple sclerosis, in Mims CA, Cruzner ML, Kelly RE (eds): *Viruses and Demyelinating Diseases.* New York, Academic Press, 1983, pp 155–165.

Waksman BH, Reynolds WE: Multiple sclerosis as a disease of immune regulation. *Proc Soc Exp Biol Med* **175:**282–294, 1984.

Walker DL, Padgett BL, Zu Rhein GM, *et al:* Human parvovirus (JC): Induction of brain tumors in hamsters. *Science* **181:**674–676, 1973.

White FA, Ishaq M, Stoner GL, *et al:* JC virus DNA is present in many human brain samples from patients without progressive multifocal leukoencephalopathy. *J Virol* **66:**5726–5734, 1992.

Zu Rhein GM: Association of papova-virions with a human demyelinating disease (multiple focal leukoencephalopathy), *Prog Med Virol* **11:**185–247, 1969.

Zu Rhein GM, Chow SM: Particles resembling papovavirus in human demyelinating disease. *Science* **148:**1477–1479, 1965.

5

Viruses and Cancer

The obstacles in establishing a possible etiological role of a virus in a human cancer include (1) the long "incubation" period between exposure to the suspected agent and the development of the disease; (2) the relatively low incidence of most cancers, which makes prospective studies almost impossible because of the large number of persons who must be kept under observation; (3) the possibility that cancer may result as a consequence of a reactivated viral infection years later rather than as a direct consequence of a primary infection; (4) the widespread and ubiquitous nature of the viruses under greatest suspicion of oncogenicity; (5) the probable role of infectious, environmental and/or genetic cofactors in producing cancer in concert with the virus or in a sequence in which the virus is the initiator and the cofactors are the promoters of tumor growth and the possibility that both of these factors may finally operate through the activation of oncogenes already present in the cell; (6) the difficulty in reproducing the malignancy in an experimental animal; and (7) the ethical impossibility of deliberately trying to reproduce the tumor in human experimentation (Evans, 1982; Evans and Mueller, 1990; Mueller *et al.*, 1993). In addition, there are many epidemiological biases and pitfalls in determining whether any exposure to a potential carcinogen, whether it be a virus, chemical, X-ray, or other agent, represents merely an association between the suspected cause and the malignancy, or a valid causal connection. These issues are discussed in Chapter 10 dealing with occupational exposures and legal proof of causality.

In animals, evidence implicating viruses as the cause of cancer in several species has been well established, even though cofactors are often needed to produce the tumor. Both RNA and DNA viruses have been implicated, as well as certain parasites. A list of some of these agents is given in Table 5.1. Most prominent in the list are certain herpesviruses of animals that are capable of inducing cancers in certain animals under defined conditions. The tumors include Marek's lymphoproliferative disease in chickens (Payne, 1972), Lucke's adenocarcinoma in leopard frogs (Lucke, 1938; Granoff, 1972), and herpes saimiri and herpes ateles viruses in monkeys (Deinhardt, 1974; Ablashi *et al.*, 1976). In addition, a retrovirus has been shown to produce a leukemia in cats (Essex *et al,*

Table 5.1
Some Viruses Producing Cancer in Animals

Feline leukemia virus in cats
Herpes ateles virus in monkeys
Herpes saimiri virus in monkeys
Lucke's virus producing adenocarcinoma of kidney in leopard frogs
Marek's virus producing a lymphoproliferative disease in chickens
Peking duck virus causing cancer of the liver
Rous sarcoma virus of chickens
Woodchuck hepatitis virus producing liver cancer

1977). Both Marek's disease and feline leukemia represent good working models for the pathogenesis of human cancers. Both represent the rare occurrence of cancer in a common and ubiquitous infection. In Marek's disease, infection occurs very early in life and is highly contagious. The requirements for malignancy include infection in the first 24 hours of life and a particular genetic susceptibility. The incidence of the subsequent tumor varies from 10 to 40% depending on the genetic stock of the chicken. These epidemiological leads have pointed the way to prevention: (1) removal of the newborn chick from the infected mother immediately at birth (exposure to the virus at a later date will result in infection but without the risk of the tumor); (2) selection of genetically resistant stocks of chicken; (3) vaccination of the newborn chick prior to exposure to the virus (Payne, 1972). This latter method has been most widely used and either a turkey herpesvirus or an attenuated strain of Marek's herpesvirus can be used; the turkey virus will not provide complete protection against later infection with natural Marek's herpesvirus but will protect against tumor development. From the standpoint of causation, it is clear that the agent can be isolated from the infected animal, grown in culture, and reproduce the tumor in another susceptible chicken, but the precise genetic and temporal aspects of the natural process must be fulfilled, i.e., cofactors are critical elements in causation. The prevention of tumors in Marek's disease by the administration of a virus vaccine very early in life also provides strong support favoring causation of this tumor by the virus (Evans, 1982). Similarly, evidence of vaccine-induced protection against herpes-associated tumors of monkeys has been reported (Ablashi et al., 1976). The feline leukemia model, so well studied by Essex and associates at· the Harvard School of Public Health, also provides insight into human oncogenetic processes (Essex et al., 1977). Finally, the woodchuck hepatitis virus (WHV) is a good model for human hepatocellular carcinoma in its pathogenesis: it proceeds from an acute hepatitis to a cirrhosis to liver cancer (Gerin et al., 1983).

In humans, the major candidate agents for causing malignant diseases are:

(1) the Epstein–Barr herpesvirus (EBV) as related to African Burkitt's lymphoma, to nasopharyngeal cancer, to acute B-cell lymphoblastic sarcoma, to B-cell tumors (especially of the brain) in patients with AIDS and in other natural, drug-induced, or genetically predisposed immunodeficiency states, such as post-transplant patients, the X-linked lymphoproliferative syndrome described by Purtillo *et al.* (1978), and an increasingly strong relationship with Hodgkin's disease (HD) and non-Hodgkin's lymphoma (NHL); (2) hepatitis B virus (HBV) in relation to primary hepatocellular carcinoma (HCC); (3) human T-cell leukemia virus, type I (HTLV-I) in the causation of acute T-cell leukemias; (4) human papillomavirus (HPV) types 16 and 18 in pathogenesis of cervical cancer, along with herpesvirus type 2 (HSV-2) as a possible cofactor (Evans and Mueller, 1990).

The general evidence relating these agents causally to the tumors with which they are associated are listed in Table 5.2. The molecular evidence has been reviewed by Zur Hausen (1991a,b). For most candidate agents, the associa-

Table 5.2
Evidence Relating a Putative Virus to a Human Cancer[a]

Epidemiological
1. The geographic distribution of infection with the virus should be similar to that of the tumor with which it is associated when adjusted for the age of infection and the presence of cofactors known to be important in tumor development
2. The presence of the viral marker (high antibody titers or antigenemia) should be higher in cases than in matched controls in the same geographic setting, as shown in case–control studies.
3. The viral marker should *precede* the tumor, and a significantly higher incidence of the tumor should follow in persons with the marker than in those without it, as shown in prospective studies.
4. Prevention of infection with the virus (vaccination) or control of the host's response to it (such as delaying the time of infection) should decrease the incidence of the tumor.

Virological
1. The virus should be able to transform human cells *in vitro* into malignant ones.
2. The viral genome or DNA should be demonstrated in tumor cells and not in normal cells.
3. The virus should be able to induce the tumor in a susceptible experimental animal and neutralization of the virus prior to injection should prevent development of the tumor.

[a]From Evans and Mueller (1990).

tion depends on epidemiological, virological, and serological evidence, the ability of the virus to transform human cells into continually proliferating or malignant forms, the experimental reproduction of the tumor in a laboratory animal, and finally, the prevention of the tumor with a vaccine prepared from the candidate agent. The rapid advances in molecular biology are also contributing information of a causal nature, especially work with oncogenes, and new techniques such as polymerase chain reaction (PCR) that demonstrate viral DNA in tumor cells. Inclusion of these lines of molecular evidence will be needed in future criteria for viruses in the causation of human cancer.

Indeed, Zur Hausen (1991a) has published such criteria. These are: (1) regular presence and persistence of nucleic acid of the virus or of a related type in cells of specific malignant tumors; (2) induction of proliferative changes upon transfection of the respective genome or parts thereof in corresponding tissue cells; (3) demonstration that the induction of these changes and the malignant phenotype of the respective tumor cells depend on the functions exerted by the persisting viral DNA; (4) epidemiologic evidence that infections with the respective virus represent risk factors for tumor development. It is clear that cancer is a complicated multistage process with many factors from the molecular to the cellular to the immunological, all playing a role in the final appearance of a cancer cell. One of the major problems in using any of the risk markers associated with a given agent is to show that the risk factor *preceded* the tumor, and therefore *might* be a causal factor, rather than the factor being the result of the tumor itself or of the immunosuppressive drugs used in its therapy. A number of malignancies are also appearing in HIV-infected persons as part of the acquired immunodeficiency syndrome (AIDS). One of these is Kaposi's sarcoma, which was a hallmark of the syndrome in homosexuals/bisexuals and is uncommon in other risk groups such as intravenous drug users, posttransfusion recipients, hemophiliacs, and perinatal infections. It appears quite early in AIDS and does not seem to be the consequence of immunodeficiency. Rather, some other factor, such as another virus, is suspected, especially one transmitted during sexual activity. The practice of "rimming," in which an active partner runs his tongue around the anus of his partner, has been associated in one unconfirmed report with an increased risk of Kaposi's sarcoma, and this suggests that some agent transmissible by the fecal–oral route may be involved. Inhalation of amyl (or other form of) nitrate is also believed by some to be a risk factor, but other studies have not supported this (Biggar, 1990). Other tumors of the lymphoma group appear in the wake of immunodeficiency as the life of the patient is prolonged by AZT. These include B-cell tumors of the brain, which are all EBV-related and monoclonal. Non-Hodgkin's lymphoma is the major lymphoma appearing in AIDS patients. Some one-third are EBV-related and some show chromosomal shifts (chromosome 8 to 22). Typical Burkitt-like lymphomas appear in chromosomal translocation and c-*myc* activation and p53 repression, but only

30% show EBV in the tumor cells (Levine and Blattner, 1992; Rabkin and Biggar, 1991). These tumors are unrelated to the nature of the HIV risk group involved. As to causation, HIV is clearly not the direct cause but sets the immunodeficiency stage for their development. The presence of the EBV genome in many of them strongly suggests that this virus is involved in the pathogenesis of the tumor, although the possibility exists that EBV is simply reactivated in the presence of immunodeficiency and that the tumor cell is permissive to entry of the virus.

The evidence involved in the association of naturally occurring virus-related tumors will now be reviewed.

Burkitt's Lymphoma

One of the strongest relationships of a virus to a human tumor is that of EBV to African Burkitt's lymphoma (BL). This tumor was described in 1958 by Denis Burkitt (Figure 5.1), an English missionary surgeon, and its epidemiology described by him in 1962 (Burkitt, 1958, 1962). The candidate causative agent, EBV, was isolated from tumor cells in 1964 by A. M. Epstein (see Figure 3.4) and his associates (Epstein et al., 1964).

Case–control studies have clearly shown an increase in a variety of EBV antibodies in BL as compared with controls, but whether this occurred after the tumor or preceded it was not known, and this evidence depended on prospective cohort studies to establish the temporal relationship. However, the challenge of establishing immunological evidence of causation of EBV in BL with prospective studies, as used for infectious mononucleosis (Hallee et al., 1974), was a formidable one because of the low incidence of the cancer, about 8–10 per 100,000 even in highly endemic tumor areas, the requirement for a large population group whose sera had to be tested, and the need for clinical surveillance for the occurrence of the tumor over a long period of time in settings where medical and diagnostic facilities are inadequate. Despite these difficulties, a massive prospective serological study of about 43,000 children in the West Nile District of Africa was launched in 1971 and a follow-up has now been carried out over 7 years (de The et al., 1978; Geser et al., 1982). Fifteen cases of BL have occurred in children for whom serum samples prior to diagnosis were available. EBV-VCA-IgG antibody was already found to be present in the sera collected at the start of the observation period from all of these cases prior to the appearance of the tumor but was of higher titer in children later developing BL than in normal children bled at the same time who did not develop the tumor. The evidence is given in Table 5.3. A titer at least twice that of the normal children carried with it a 30-fold increased risk of the subsequent development of BL. BL also developed in two children whose initial antibody level was not elevated. EBV genome was

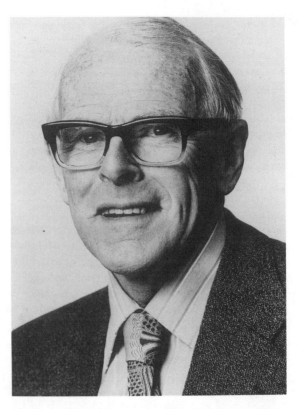

Figure 5.1. Dr. Denis P. Burkitt (1911–), missionary surgeon, Hartwell Cottage, Gloucester, England.

also demonstrated in five of seven biopsy specimens taken after the tumor had developed and in these, other EBV antibodies also rose. However, the genome was absent in the two cases with initially normal EBV-VCA-IgG antibody titers. While those children with initially high EBV titers represented the group at highest risk to subsequent development of BL, only a small proportion actually developed the tumor. Thus, while high EBV antibodies were a risk factor, they were neither necessary nor sufficient to produce the tumor. EBV can be considered an *initiating* event that leads to B-lymphocyte proliferation (immortalization) which is further stimulated by malaria both by a direct mitogenic action and by interference with the T-cell control of EBV multiplication. This can be regarded as a *promoting* factor (Evans, 1985). In the course of these rapidly multiplying B cells, a chromosomal shift from chromosome 8 to 14 occurs (sometimes to 2 or 22) that carries with it an oncogene, c-*myc*, which then becomes activated (or derepressed) in its new location and a single malignant clone of b cells arises whose growth ultimately leads to BL (Evans, 1982; Evans and de The, 1989). The fact that an EBV antigen called EB nuclear antigen type-1 (EBNA-1) is the only one expressed on the surface of the BL cell and is not recognized by T lymphocytes may be the reason for the uncontrolled growth of this cell (McGrath, 1992). The evidence relating EBV to BL is summarized in Table 5.4. The presence of the EBV genome in every African BL cell is strong circumstantial evidence of association, fulfilling the first Henle–Koch postulate. The tumor is monoclonal, suggesting that EBV must have been present in the malignantly transformed cell at the start. The process is much more complicated, however. A current concept of pathogenesis is that the rapid B-cell proliferation leads to a chromosomal shift from chromosome 8 to 14 in some 70% of cases, and from 8 to 2 or 22 in other cases. This translocation carries with it an immuno-globulin gene and the c-*myc* oncogene. In its new location the oncogene becomes derepressed or activated, and this event results in the appearance of a monoclonal malignant cell that proliferates and leads to BL. A protein, p53, that controls the proliferation of malignant cells is also repressed (McGrath, 1992). This complicated web of events indicates that EBV is but one of several factors involved in the oncogenic process and probably not an essential one. Indeed, the formation of BL on histological grounds occurs at a low level of endemicity. The occurrence of infection with EBV and malaria early in life may greatly accelerate

Table 5.3
Results of Prospective Study of Burkitt's Lymphoma (BL) in Uganda[a]

43,000 children bled and followed initially over 5 years.

14 developed BL (about 7 per 100,000 per year).

All cases had EBV antibody in the pretumor sera.

12 or 13 of the histologically proven cases of BL had VCA-IgG antibody titers as high or higher than age/sex/locality-matched controls.

The increased risk of developing BL was estimated to be 30 times in children who had antibody levels two dilutions or more above the geometric mean titer of the corresponding normal population standardized for age, sex, and locality.

The presence of EBV DNA and EBNA was established in 9 of 10 cases from whom frozen biopsies were available.

Antibodies to herpes simplex, cytomegalovirus, and measles virus were not elevated in the pre-BL sera as compared to controls, nor were other EBV antibodies, such as early (EA) and nuclear antigens (EBNA).

The final results indicated a high degree of significance ($p = 0.002$) between the VCA antibody titers in pre-BL sera as compared to matched controls.

[a]Derived from data in de The *et al.* (1978).

Table 5.4
Evidence Relating EBV to African Burkitt's Lymphoma and to Nasopharyngeal Carcinoma[a]

Seroepidemiological	EBV antibody elevated in over 80% of both. EBV IgG antibody precedes diagnosis of BL. IgA antibody is characteristic of nasopharyngeal carcinoma and may precede diagnosis, at least in some cases.
Virological	EBV genome or DNA regularly present in tumor cells of both. EBV causes malignant transformation of B cells *in vitro* and lymphoma in cotton-top marmosets and owl monkeys. Nasopharyngeal carcinoma has not been reproduced with EBV laboratory animals.
Cofactors	Holoendemic malaria plays key role in African Burkitt's lymphoma. Chromosomal translocations and c-*myc* activation are required for Burkitt's lymphoma. Genetic susceptibility and nitrosamines are important for nasopharyngeal carcinoma.

[a]Derived from Evans and Mueller (1990).

B-cell proliferation and the chance that BL will develop (Miller, 1974). However, the reproduction of a malignant lymphoma in cotton-top marmosets (Shope *et al.*, 1973) and in owl monkeys (Epstein *et al.*, 1973) with EBV-infected lymphocytes or semipurified virus shows the malignant potential of EBV and moves toward fulfillment of the third postulate of Henle–Koch in the relationship of EBV to African BL.

In the United States, where infection with EBV in infancy is uncommon and where malaria is absent, only about one third of the BL cases are EBV-related. The evidence for this is derived from EBV antibody studies carried out on 119 cases reported to the National Burkitt Registry at the National Cancer Institute, in which only 25–30% showed elevated EBV-VCA-IgG antibody titers and/or had EBV genome demonstrable in the tumor tissue. Some 45% had normal EBV antibody levels and 19% had no demonstrable EBV antibody at all, indicating that infection with the virus never occurred (Evans, 1982). Some factor other than EBV must, therefore, be an initiator of the B-cell proliferation, chromosomal shift, and c-*myc* activation in those cases with normal or absent EBV antibodies. EBV genome was found in tumor cells in 25–30% of cases so studied at the National Burkitt Registry. It should be emphasized that 19% lacked EBV antibody altogether, indicating a different etiology (Evans, 1985).

In summary, EBV is implicated as the probable initiating factor in the majority of BL cases occurring in highly endemic areas where malaria acts as a promoter. In addition to these factors, a chromosomal shift and a resulting activation of c-*myc* and perhaps other oncogenes are necessary for the malignant process to occur. This complex web of interacting factors indicates that EBV is neither a necessary nor a sufficient cause of BL, but plays a role in initiating the process in very young children in certain areas of the world (Evans and de The, 1989).

Nasopharyngeal Carcinoma

EBV has also been implicated as a risk factor in nasopharyngeal carcinoma (NPC), which occurs worldwide in adults but with much higher incidence in persons of Oriental birth, especially in the southern area of mainland China. The antibody elevations and the presence of EBV genome in the tumor cells are almost identical to those found in African BL, but no chromosomal shift has been demonstrated and the tumor has not been reproduced in experimental animals (de The *et al.*, 1989). Large, planned prospective studies, such as carried out in Africa for BL, have not been performed for NPC. However, mass screening tests for the presence of EBV-VCA-IgA antibody, which is a characteristic marker of the tumor, have been done on large numbers of adults in high-risk populations in southern China. These tests have shown that the antibody is a strong risk marker for the presence of NPC. For example, 117 persons with IgA antibody were detected in the screening of some 50,000 persons, and subsequent examination of the antibody-positive group revealed 19 cases of NPC (Zeng *et al.*, 1982). Follow-up studies also showed that two cases later developed NPC. The presence of IgA prior to tumor development has also been reported by Ho *et al.* (1978). Such evidence suggests that EBV-IgA may be a predictive risk marker but it does not *establish* causation.

The individuals in these studies were followed on the basis of having EBV-VCA-IgA antibody, which does not eliminate the possibility that persons without prior elevation of this antibody might also develop NPC. Indeed, we have recently failed to find elevated EBV-VCA-IgA antibody titers in preillness sera from seven persons who developed NPC 26 to 154 months later (Chan *et al.*, 1991). No elevations for EBV-EA-D, EBV-EA-R, or EBNA were found as compared with matched controls. However, the geometric mean titer of EBV-VCA-IgG antibody was elevated somewhat above matched control sera (88.3 versus 75.5, $p < 0.05$), especially among Asian individuals. In this small series, our results do not indicate that EBV reactivation precedes NPC in the period during which the preillness sera were collected. This is in contrast to our findings in prediagnostic sera from Hodgkin's disease (Evans and Comstock, 1981; Mueller *et al.*, 1989) and non-Hodgkin's lymphoma (Mueller *et al.*, 1991).

Other factors such as eating dried fish containing nitrosamines and certain genetic traits (HLA-2, SIN) have also been incriminated as risk factors, perhaps in increasing the susceptibility of the nasopharyngeal epithelium to infection by EBV. At this time, it is not clear if EBV infection of nasopharyngeal cells is a necessary prelude to NPC or occurs subsequent to the development of the tumor.

Except for the varying presence of elevated EBV-VCA-IgA antibody titers in prediagnostic sera, no geographic variations in the pattern of EBV antibodies or of EBV genome in tumor tissues have been found once the tumor has been diagnosed, in contrast to variable patterns in African and American BL (Evans and de The, 1989). EBV has a very strong association with NPC.

Hodgkin's Disease

EBV has also been implicated in the pathogenesis of at least some cases of Hodgkin's disease (HD). The evidence for this is that 30–40% of HD cases worldwide have elevated antibody titers to several EBV antigens at the time of diagnosis as compared with age- and sex-matched controls, and these have been shown to precede immunosuppressive therapy for the tumor (Mueller, 1987). However, it was not known if the antibody elevations resulted from the tumor itself or preceded it, and therefore might be a risk factor in the pathogenesis of the tumor. A pilot study suggested they did precede diagnosis (Evans and Comstock, 1981). Recently, a massive prospective study of 240,000 normal persons who were bled in the past and then followed in tumor or hospital registries for the development of the tumor revealed 43 confirmed cases of HD. Sera from these cases were then tested for various EBV antibodies and cytomegalovirus and compared with 196 age- and sex-matched controls who had been bled at the same time and who did not develop cancer during the subsequent observation period (Mueller *et al.*, 1989). The results showed significantly elevated EBV antibody titers in persons subsequently developing the tumor than in controls. These altered antibody patterns were most common 3 to 5 years preceding the appearance of HD. Interpretation of these findings was not clear initially. It now seems probable that EBV plays a direct role in the development of many cases of HD, as evidenced by the recent demonstration of EBV DNA in Reed–Sternberg cells of biopsy tissue or paraffin-fixed tissues by *in situ* hybridization or polymerase chain reaction (PCR) (Hamilton-Dutoit *et al.*, 1989; Weiss *et al.*, 1989; Herbst *et al.*, 1990, 1991). In tissues from 150 cases of HD examined by PCR, Herbst *et al.* (1990) found EBV DNA in 50%, which was located in the Reed–Sternberg cells and confined to tumor tissue. Using these sensitive techniques, about 50% of all recently tested material from HD showed evidence of the virus or its DNA in tumor cells, the percentage depending on the tumor type, and being as high as 90% in the mixed cellularity form. These findings do not necessarily prove that EBV caused the tumor, but its presence in so many cells and in so many cases is very strong evidence of this when considered along with the prospective evidence of raised EBV antibody titers prior to diagnosis (Mueller *et al.*, 1989). A second possible explanation of the pretumor antibody findings is that EBV may set the immunological stage for the action of some other oncogenic agent. Third, the elevated EBV antibody levels could simply be a marker for the reactivation of the virus by some other virus, or environmental or genetic factor, that disturbs the immune system. The mounting molecular evidence favors the first explanation.

Non-Hodgkin's Lymphoma

As mentioned earlier in this discussion, non-Hodgkin's lymphoma (NHL) is increasing in AIDS patients owing in part to their longer life spans under AZT therapy. This tumor also occurs in patients immunosuppressed by drugs used for organ transplants, in cases of acquired and congenital immunodeficiency, in the X-linked lymphoproliferative syndrome, and there is suggestive evidence of an increase in "spontaneous" cases. In these NHL patients, the involvement of EBV is suggested by the presence of EBV DNA in tumor tissue (Ho *et al.*, 1985; Hanto *et al.*, 1981; List *et al.*, 1987) and by altered serological patterns to EBV (Ferrell *et al.*, 1981; Masucci *et al.*, 1984; Birx *et al.*, 1983; Lindemalm *et al.*, 1983). My colleagues and I have carried out a prospective cohort study to determine if such altered EBV antibody patterns preceded the diagnosis of NHL and were a risk factor in its development (Mueller *et al.*, 1991), in the same way that we have shown for pre-HD sera (Mueller *et al.*, 1989). From sera collected from 240,000 persons who were followed for the development of virus-related malignancies, 104 cases of NHL were identified. The blood had been collected an average of 63 months prior to diagnosis. Their EBV antibody patterns were compared with 259 matched controls. Higher EBV IgG and IgM antibody titers to the viral capsid antigen were found in sera from prediagnostic individuals as compared with controls, with relative risks of subsequently developing NHL of 2.4 and 5.1, respectively. Antibody titers to EBNA, however, were lower than controls (RR = 0.5). These antibody patterns resembled those found at the time of tumor occurrence, and were similar to those found in AIDS patients and others with evidence of immunodeficiency. They are in contrast to those found in pre-HD sera, in that IgM antibody was elevated and EBNA was low in NHL and not in HD. This suggests a different pathogenetic mechanism.

Lymphomas and Other Malignancies in AIDS Patients

The common tumors reported in patients with AIDS include Kaposi's sarcoma, Burkitt's lymphoma, lymphomas of the brain, Hodgkin's disease, non-

Hodgkin's lymphoma, leukemias, and hepatomas (Biggar, 1990; Rabkin and Biggar, 1991). Kaposi's sarcoma, a hallmark of AIDS, occurs primarily in homosexual men. It is also being observed in men who are HIV-antibody-negative. It may be related to certain sexual practices such as "rimming," in which oral–anal contact occurs. It is believed that an unknown agent, possibly a virus transmitted by sexual intercourse, and possibly present in the stool of HIV-infected persons (and perhaps in the absence of HIV infection), is a causal factor in this tumor. Use of amyl nitrate to increase sexual response has been incriminated by some studies, but not by others, as a risk factor for Kaposi's sarcoma.

Lymphomas, of a variety of types other than HD, have shown a marked increase in AIDS patients as compared to the general population, probably related to the longer survival of patients treated with AZT. In a study of 97,258 AIDS patients reported to the Centers for Disease Control, 2824 cases of non-HD lymphomas (2.9%) were identified (Beral *et al.*, 1991). These included 1686 cases of immunoblastic sarcoma, 545 cases of primary lymphomas of the brain, and 590 cases of BL (a tumor not normally associated with immunosuppression). Each occurred more commonly in whites than in blacks. Unlike Kaposi's sarcoma, no predominant association with sexual practices was observed. While several causal agents were implicated in the pathogenesis of these tumors, EBV was the predominant one. From other studies, almost all primary lymphomas of the brain in AIDS patients have been found to contain EBV DNA in the tumor cells, about half of the cases of immunoblastic sarcoma, and one fifth of the cases of BL (Rabkin and Biggar, 1991; Levine and Blattner, 1992). The association with EBV DNA has been more common in these AIDS patients than in other patients with these lymphomas occurring in the United States. In African BL, however, over 95% are EBV-related and appear to represent the consequences of a primary infection with the virus rather than the reactivated infection in HIV-immunosuppressed patients. While the pathogenesis of these EBV-related B-cell lymphomas in AIDS patients is not clear, it seems likely that the virus plays an important role in the causation of a substantial percentage of them, but that other viruses or agents can result in the same histological type in other cases.

Hepatitis B Virus (HBV) and Hepatocellular Carcinoma (HCC)

The strongest causal evidence that a virus "causes" a human cancer is probably the relationship between HBV and HCC. The main epidemiological marker in this instance is the presence of HBV antigenemia and the major host factor is infection early in life, which increases the risk of lifelong persistence of the antigen in over 60% as compared with 10% in older children and adults. The causal relationships between the virus and the tumor were well summarized in

Table 5.5
Relationship of Hepatitis B Virus (HBV) to Hepatocellular Carcinoma (HCC)[a]

1. The geographic distribution of hepatocellular cancer correlates closely with hepatitis B (HBsAg) Antegenemia.
2. In areas of high HCC incidence, HBsAg antigenemia can be detected in 37 to 80% of cancer patients, a frequency 10 to 15 times higher than in controls.
3. In high-incidence areas, the prevalence of antibody to HBsAg is about half that of healthy controls.
4. Only 5% of African and 26% of American patients with HCC lack demonstrable evidence of current or past HBV infection.
5. The relative risk of past exposure to HBV is 1.0 to 1.5 times that of controls in high-incidence areas and 10 to 15 times that of controls in low-incidence areas.
6. In one study, 82% of nonalcoholic cirrhosis patients had at least one HBV marker.
7. Mothers of HCC patients were HBsAg positive four times more frequently than fathers; in control mothers and fathers, the rates were the same.

[a]From Szmuness (1978)

1978 by the late W. Szmuness (1978) as shown in Table 5.5. It is based on the parallel association of HBV antigenemia and HCC in different geographic areas and the consistency of this association in both high- and low-incidence areas, albeit with a different magnitude of difference; on the higher frequency of antigen in mothers of children who later developed HCC than in fathers; and on various case–control comparisons demonstrating the greater prevalence of antigenemia in HCC patients than in controls or in the general population of that area. These seroepidemiological data have subsequently been strongly reinforced by a massive prospective study of 22,707 males in Taiwan followed an average of 6.2 years for the development of HCC in HBV-antigen-negative and -positive male government workers, which was carried out by Beasley, Hwang, and associates (Beasley *et al.*, 1981). The initial results indicated that the risk of dying from HCC in antigen-positive men was over 200 times greater than that for antigen-negative men. HCC developed in 113 of 3454 originally antigen-positive men (1 in 30.6 men) as compared with only 3 in 19,253 initially antigen-negative men (1 in 6418 men). The incidence of HCC remained essentially constant during the observation period, indicating a continuous process of tumor development. While cirrhosis was also much more common in antigen-positive men, it was not essential for the development of HCC. Indeed, none of the 30 antigen-negative

Table 5.6
Tawian Prospective Study: Hepatocellular Carcinoma (HCC) Incidence and Relative Risk through December 31, 1986[a,b]

Recruitment status	HCC	Population at risk	HCC/100,000	RR
HBsAg+	152	3,454	494.5	
HBsAg−	9	19,253	5.3	98.4
Total	161	22,707	79.7	

[a]From Beasley (1987).
[b]Values provided for 8.9 years for follow-up; 95% confidence interval on RR is 50.2–193.0.

men who had cirrhosis at the start of the study developed HCC. This supports the concept that HBV, and not cirrhosis, is the causal risk factor in HCC. In further follow-up of these persons over a period of 11.5 years, as shown in Table 5.6, the relative risk dropped to 98.4 but is still very impressive (Beasley, 1990). The suggested pathogenesis is that HBV infection early in life results in persistent antigenemia in about 95%, which leads to HCC; some individuals also develop cirrhosis prior to HCC. The lesson in prevention from these data is that if HBV is the true and necessary cause, then HBV immunization must be given in the first 2 weeks of life if HCC is to be prevented. The risk of HBV infection to the newborn is largely dependent on the presence of "e" antigen in the infected mother. Infection in adult life results in a persistent antigenemia is only about 10% of these adults, so that the risk of HCC is very much less among those infected. It should be noted that in this prospective study, as well as in the review of many case–control studies by Szmuness (1978), not all cases of HCC have demonstrable evidence of present or past HBV infection. In Africa and other high-incidence areas, the great majority do have antigenemia (90%), but in low-incidence areas such as America, only 25% do. This situation is similar to that of EBV and BL in Africa and America. In both instances the strong association with the putative agents in Africa is due to the early age of infection; in America, infection usually occurs at a much later age with both agents, and other causes ultimately lead to a morphologically similar cancer. The other causes of HCC are not known but aflatoxin, present in moldy grain, is a suspected cause or cofactor in certain areas, such as China, where the risk of HBV-associated HCC increases with the degree of exposure to aflatoxin (Beasley, 1990). The mechanism of action of aflatoxin in HCC is unknown, but there is suggestive evidence that it may alter a gene called p53 located on chromosome 17, which is intimately involved in cell growth when a mutation occurs. This changes it from its usual role in suppression of growth to one of growth enhancement. Mutations in this gene, either congenital or acquired, may lie behind several malignancies in collaboration with other cancer-regulatory genes (*The New York Times,* 1991).

Recent evidence has also incriminated hepatitis C virus (HCV) in cirrhosis and HCC in cases not due to HBV. This virus was previously called non-A, non-B virus, parenteral type (Kiyosawa *et al.,* 1990; Evans and Mueller, 1990). With methods of antibody detection at hand in commercial kits, and with the development of a nested polymerase chain reaction to detect antigen in blood and tissues, the evidence for its role in acute and viral hepatitis and in cirrhosis and cancer should mount rapidly. It is already clear that infective virus can coexist in the serum in the presence of antibody, posing a strong hazard to recipients of HCV-antibody-positive blood. HCV is now established as the major cause of post-transfusion hepatitis in developed countries where screening for HBV has eliminated most cases due to that virus.

With regard to the serological and epidemiological evidence relating HBV to HCC, there is direct virological evidence that HBV is involved in the pathogenesis of HCC in that HBV DNA has been demonstrated frequently in HCC tissue (Melnick, 1989). However, the tumor has not been experimentally reproduced in nonhuman primates, although similar hepatitis viruses of woodchucks and of Peking ducks result in liver tumors in their own species. A hepatitis B vaccine is now available in several forms and has been shown to be highly effective in protecting against HBV infection (Hadler and Margolis, 1989). It is now widely used in developed countries in high-risk groups, albeit inadequately to stem the increasing incidence of the infection, especially in homosexuals and I.V. drug abusers. Large-scale field trials in newborn infants are now in progress in several high-incidence areas of the world for HCC to determine if prevention of HBV infection early in life will protect against the development of HCC in adult life. The logistics of giving the vaccine prior to infection, and the inability, costwise, to give immune globulin to provide immediate protection until the vaccine takes effect, result in an estimated 70% protection efficacy against HBV infection. Such trials are being carried out by several national governments in collaboration with the World Health Organization. If such trials are successful in preventing or greatly reducing that proportion of HCC attributable to HBV, then a very strong link in causal association will have been forged. At that time, I think one will be justified in stating that HBV is a necessary and sufficient cause of a substantial proportion of HCC cases in developing countries.

Genital Herpes, Papillomaviruses, and Cervical Cancer

The relationship between herpes simplex virus, type 2, and cervical cancer is based on serological and virological evidence similar to that outlined for EBV and

Table 5.7
Evidence Relating HSV-2 to Cervical Cancer[a]

Seroepidemiological

1. HSV-2 (VCA) antibody more common in cases than in controls: 20 of 30 studies showed differences.
2. Antibody to Ag4 antigen: 85% positive in invasive cancer, 65% in *in situ* cancer, 7% noncancer.
3. Antibody to nonvirion, HSV-TAA antigen: 85% positive in cancer of cervix; noncancer 4%.
4. Prospective data: higher cancer incidence in HSV-2-antibody-positive persons than in HSV-negative persons.

Virological

1. Herpesvirus antigens present in some tumor cells.
2. Isolation of HSV from culture of cervical cells.
3. Cell transformation by HSV in hamsters.

---

[a]From Evans (1982).

BL. However, the evidence of causation is far less convincing. The available information was summarized in 1982 (Evans, 1982) and is reproduced in Table 5.7.

The major reasons for not obtaining valid data have been difficult technical problems in the laboratory concerning differentiation between the widely prevalent herpes type 1 antibody and the type 2 antibody incriminated in cervical cancer. Since infection with HSV-1 usually occurs early in life, and that with HSV-2 at an age when sexual transmission of the agent begins, it is usually necessary to identify HSV-1 antibody in the presence of HSV-2 antibody. Recent technical developments in differential antibody tests, such as the immunoblot and other methods, now provide much more accurate differentiation (Nahmias and Josey, 1989) between the two types, but all of the earlier seroepidemiological data were plagued by this problem. Furthermore, since HSV-1 infection is increasingly being transmitted by sexual means, it may be more appropriate to speak of "genital herpes" without reference to the type.

Different workers have used different serological methods. There are cross-reactions between the two antibodies, and HSV type 2 almost never occurs in the absence of type 1 antibody. Just as an association has been found between EBV and African but not American BL, so geographic differences in HSV type 2 and cervical cancer also exist, but on a much wider scale and without apparent reason, which is unlike the presence of early EBV infection and of holoendemic malaria to explain geographic variations in BL. It appears that there is a five- to tenfold higher relative risk of invasive cervical cancer in individuals with HSV-2 antibody as compared with those without antibody in Brussels, Copenhagen, and Atlanta (in Negroes) but a relatively low risk or no increased risk in Israel, Auckland, and Yugoslavia (Melnick *et al.*, 1989); quite marked variations have even been observed within the same geographic area. Epidemiologically, the most striking association of cervical cancer is not with herpesvirus *per se* but with sexual intercourse. The age of onset of sexual activity, the number of sexual partners, the frequency of the act, and a history of smoking are all positively correlated with the risk of cervical cancer in women. Smoking has been a risk factor in many studies in different geographic areas of a magnitude of about two for persons smoking over 40 cigarettes daily or smoking of many years duration, particularly when smoking was started early in life. Oral contraceptives have been incriminated as a risk factor in some studies, but this has not been too impressive when controlled for sexual activity. In the male, a history of multiple sexual partners and of penile cancer also increases the risk in his sexual partner. A venereally transmitted oncogenic agent other than HSV-2 in some areas of the world (or even in the United States) has not been fully excluded; several agents, including viruses and chemicals, may be able to induce cancer, either singly or in concert.

With both EBV and HSV-2, it is clear that the age, geographic location, and the behavioral, genetic, and immunological characteristics of the infected host play a decisive role in the development of cancer with agents as prevalent and ubiquitous as the herpesviruses. In my opinion, and that of Rawls *et al.* (1977), who drew up five criteria for causation, the available evidence does not support a firm causal relationship at the present time. As pointed out later in this discussion, HSV may only operate as a cofactor with papillomavirus. The most impressive negative evidence in my mind are the two large-scale prospective seroepidemiological studies carried out by Adam *et al.* (1985) in Houston, Texas and by Vonka *et al.* (1984) in Prague, Czechoslovakia using modernized methods for distinguishing between HSV-1 and HSV-2 antibody. In neither study could an increased risk for the development of cervical cancer be found in women possessing HSV-2 antibody as compared with women lacking this antibody. Both studies employed good epidemiological, laboratory, and ascertainment techniques. While it is possible that methodological differences may explain the lack of association in these prospective studies as compared with the associations found in case–control studies as summarized by Melnick *et al.* (1989), they certainly weaken the HSV virus–cancer association as compared with the prospective data derived from EBV/African BL and HBV/HCC. The lack of geographic consistency in the relationship of HSV-2 and cervical cancer in many countries, the laboratory problems of reproducibility of the results of others, and even of one's own results, the failure to demonstrate HSV DNA regularly in cervical cancer tissue, and the inability to reproduce the full malignancy in experimental animals all weaken the putative association of genital herpes with cervical carcinoma.

In recent years there is increasing evidence that human papillomaviruses (HPV), especially types 16 and 18, are involved in the pathogenesis of cervical cancer (Zur Hausen, 1977, 1982, 1985, 1987, 1991a,b; Pater and Pater, 1985; Pater *et al.*, 1986; Melnick *et al.*, 1989). The evidence is primarily virological because satisfactory techniques for measuring antibody to the virus have not been worked out. Melnick (1989) has summarized the supporting observations as follows: "(1) The HPV is the only DNA-containing virus that induces benign tumors in the natural host. (2) Certain benign lesions can convert to squamous cell carcinoma. (3) Several nonhuman papillomaviruses can induce cancers in their natural hosts. (4) The HPV is epitheliotropic, and most human cancers are carcinomas." DNA sequences of HPV types 16 and 18 have been identified in cell lines from cervical cancer (Boshart *et al.*, 1984; Pater and Pater, 1985) in which the DNA has been shown to be integrated and transcriptionally active (Smotkin and Wellstein, 1986). Cloned HPV type 16 DNA or DNA extracted from a cervical cancer containing this HPV type has been shown to be capable of transforming NIH 3T3 cells *in vitro* (Yasumoto *et al.*, 1986). Evidence of the presence of papillomavirus, especially type 18, has been regularly found in higher frequency in tissues from cervical cancer than in normal tissues. For example, in a case–control study of invasive cancer in Latin America, 66% of the cases had HPV genotype 16 or 18 DNA in tissue specimens compared with 46% in control tissue (Reeves *et al.*, 1987). Infection with HPV and early age of first intercourse were found to be the major risk factors. In a survey of 9295 women in Germany undergoing cytological examinations in routine hospital examinations, de Villiers *et al.* (1987) compared the frequency of HPV infections among women with and without normal cytological findings. Of the 94% with normal smears, HPV was found in 10% among women aged 15–45 and in less than 5% of women over 50 years old. Among those with abnormal smears, representing cervical intraepithelial neoplasias I, II, and III and invasive cancer, HPV was found in 30–40% and was age dependent. The filter *in situ* hybridization method employed was said to underestimate the total HPV infection rate by a factor of 2 or 3. In other papers from this group, Zur Hausen (1985, 1986, 1987a,b, 1991a,b) has expressed the opinion that papillomavirus is a necessary but not sufficient cause of cervical cancer. Other factors such as HSV-2, or other initiating events, such as cigarette smoking, may operate as cofactors in its production. He feels that loss of intracellular control of HPV results in the expression of the papilloma gene (Zur Hausen, 1986, 1991b). More work in different laboratories is needed to confirm the important observations of Zur Hausen, but the evidence is mounting that certain strains of papillomavirus are involved in the pathogenesis of cervical and other epithelial cancers. Of great importance would be the demonstration in prospective cohort studies that HPV DNA in cervical tissues *preceded* the appearance of the malignancy, and that persons with the virus in cervical tissue were at much higher risk for subsequent development of the tumor than are those lacking the antigen, or having it at a much lower frequency. This may not be an impossible epidemiological and technical task if cells obtained during routine Pap testing can be used for a reliable determination of the presence or absence of the viral DNA. Such persons can then be followed in laboratories doing mass survey studies or through cancer registries tied in with laboratories carrying out the testing, such as large state or cancer laboratories. However, the prospective study of Adam *et al.* (1985) in Houston failed to find histological evidence of HPV infection in biopsies taken at the start of the study, either in the women who subsequently developed cervical intraepithelial neoplasia (CIN) or in those who did not. Specimens obtained later from 14 of 17 women who developed CIN I or II and from 3 of 6 women who developed CIN III had histological evidence of concurrent HPV infection. Thus, it could not be established in this study that HPV preceded CIN.

Human T-cell Leukemia Virus, Type I (HTLV-I) and T-cell Leukemia

The human T-cell leukemia/lymphoma virus, type I was first isolated by Poiesz *et al.* (1980) from patients with cutaneous T-cell leukemia. It is associated with a rare adult T-cell leukemia (Robert-Guroff and Gallo, 1983) by epidemiological and virological evidence. More recently, a strong causal association with tropical spastic paraparesis (TSP) has been identified (Bartholomew *et al.*, 1986). Other terms for the condition are Jamaican neuropathy and HTLV-I-associated myelopathy (HAM) for the Japanese cases. Involvement of the brain, of the joints, and, in Jamaica, of the skin is now being recognized as less common clinical manifestations. The virus is transmitted perinatally, mainly via breast milk, by sexual intercourse, and by blood transfusion. The epidemiological features are unusual, however, in their geographic restriction and high degree of microendemicity.

Many epidemiological studies of the prevalence of antibody to the virus have been carried out by Blattner and his associates at the National Cancer Institute as well as by Japanese investigators (Hinuma *et al.*, 1982; Tajima and Hinuma, 1982; Maeda *et al.*, 1984) as reviewed in a recent chapter by Blattner (Blattner, 1989). An excellent review of the epidemiology of HTLV-I has been written by Mueller (1991). Infection with the virus appears to occur mainly in southern Japan (antibody prevalence rates of > 20%), to some degree in the Caribbean islands and certain West African countries (rates 10–19%), and to a lesser extent (1–9%) in Australian aborigines, Florida Indians, Panama, the

Solomon islands, and Papua New Guinea (although there are some pockets of high prevalence in this latter area). Rates under 1% have been found in American blacks in the southern United States. In Africa, both humans and monkeys are infected (Hunsmann *et al.,* 1983). In Japan, prevalence rates approach 30% in some areas and there is evidence of familial clustering. However, areas very close to one another may have quite different rates, suggesting the importance of person-to-person and perinatal transmission in highly endemic areas. In addition to the high prevalence rates in southern Japan, there are also high rates in the aboriginal Ainu population of northern Japan. The data suggest that this virus is an ancient one, long present in small clusters among isolated groups.

Among those infected with the virus, the rate of occurrence of the tumor is very low, on the order of 1 in 1000. The reason why some persons develop the tumor and others do not is not known. However, the route of transmission appears to bear on the type of clinical syndrome manifested. Adult T-cell leukemia/lymphoma (ATL) is primarily associated with perinatal transmission, especially through breast milk of infected mothers, whereas TSP (HAM) is mainly associated with transfusion of infected blood. The prevalence rates in the Caribbean islands of St. Vincent, Martinique, and Barbados range from 3 to 5% (mainly in adults); the rate in Jamaica is higher. Sera from a health and serological survey carried out in Bridgetown, Barbados in 1972 by Evans *et al.* (1974) have recently been tested for antibodies to HTLV-I (Reidel *et al.,* 1989). The antibody prevalence rate was 4.3% in sera from 1012 persons; there was an age-dependent increase in prevalence, and female predominance (5.7 versus 2.2%). The only positive children were from antibody-positive mothers, suggesting transmission by vertical or perinatal routes or via breast-feeding. Transmission sexually was also strongly suggested by a 4-fold higher prevalence rate of antibody in females and a 2.6-fold higher rate in males who had a positive test for syphilis (FTA-absorbed test). Clustering in households but not in neighborhoods was seen. These epidemiological findings are in general agreement with those in other areas, but were made on sera taken in 1972, 8 years before HTLV-I was discovered. No evidence is available to indicate whether T-cell leukemias have occurred in this group but the low incidence of this leukemia among infected persons suggests that only one or two cases could have been expected. This also means that prospective cohort studies to determine the frequency of the leukemia in antibody-positive versus antibody-negative persons will require a very large population base and a careful follow-up in hospitals where a confirmatory diagnosis of the tumor can be made.

Current knowledge of the natural history of HTLV-I infection indicates that a latent state occurs after primary infection, with the apparent reservoir of infection existing in peripheral blood T lymphocytes. The virus is closely cell-bound and no circulating viral products are detectable. A protein, p40/42, called the "tax protein," (or p42), is strongly associated with the multiplication of the virus through transactivation of viral transcription (Mueller, 1991). The virus is also able to immortalize activated T-helper cells bearing a CD4 marker and Tac $^+$ (or CD25), the IL-2 receptor (Mueller 1991; Rosenblatt *et al.,* 1988). In high-incidence areas, epidemiological evidence of the causal relationship of HTLV-I infection and adult T-cell leukemia/lymphoma (ATL) is strong, in that both occur in the same geographic areas, HTLV-I antibody is present in almost all cases, and in follow-up of HTLV-I infected cases a lifetime risk of 2–5% has been estimated for the carriers, depending on the time of the initial infection. The presence of over 5% atypical lymphocytes appears to be an early marker of risk for ATL. Lower levels of atypical lymphocytosis (under 3%) have been observed in the carrier state along with polyclonally integrated HTLV-I provirus, and some level of immune dysfunction. Such suppression of immune function, with loss of PPD skin reactivity, has been a regular feature of smoldering ATL, which increases with advancing age (Mueller, 1991). In addition, the virus has transforming ability, and there is good evidence that the HTLV-I genome is present in tumor cells in an integrated fashion and that the tumor cell is monoclonal—both strong evidence of causality. Missing causal evidence is the failure thus far to reproduce the tumor in experimental animals, and of large-scale prospective cohort studies indicating the risk of ATL in HTLV-I antibody-positive and antibody-negative persons; such studies are under way in southern Japan.

Worldwide, only 80% of the cases of T-cell leukemia tested have shown a demonstrable relationship to HTLV-I, mainly by the presence of antibody, so that other causes of the leukemia probably exist. At the moment, the virus remains a very strong candidate as a major causal factor in the pathogenesis of most cases of adult T-cell leukemia and perhaps all cases of spastic tropical paraparesis (HAM). Based on recent observations of the presence of HTLV-I antibody in I.V. drug users in New Orleans (Weiss, 1989), and in several New Jersey communities, this virus and the risk of leukemia may become important possibilities in the United States in these groups, in their sexual partners, and in persons who have received their donated blood. Testing for antibody to HTLV-I has become routine in highly endemic areas, and nationally may become necessary in high-risk U.S. populations although current surveys of blood donors indicate such low general prevalence rates that such testing would not currently be cost-effective.

Summary

Viruses probably play a role in the induction of about 10% of all fatal malignancies in the United States (Doll and Peto, 1981; Evans, 1982) and a much higher percentage in developing countries, such as BL in Africa, NPC in Oriental populations, HCC in Africa and Asia, and ATL in Japan. The strength of the causal relationship is strongest for HBV and HCC and for HTLV-I and human T-cell leukemia/lymphoma. EBV plays a key role as an initiator of African BL along with malaria as a promoter in a complex web of pathogenesis that includes a chromosomal translocation, the activation of an oncogene and the suppression of p53 gene; there is increasing evidence that it plays a causal role in many cases of Hodgkin's lymphoma and some cases of non-Hodgkin's lymphoma, including the occurrence of these tumors and of primary B-cell lymphomas of the brain in AIDS patients. HPV types 16 and 18 are increasingly incriminated in the causation of cervical and other epithelial cancers, such as rectal and laryngeal. However, our limited technical ability to detect the specific presence of the virus, especially in large-scale prospective cohort epidemiological studies, its occurrence in normal tissues, and the lack of a way to measure antibody (or a poor immunologic response), all severely limit virological and epidemiological investigation. The good news is that studies of the virus–cancer relationships are yielding important advances in our understanding of the complex molecular and genetic events involved in the process of oncogenesis, and that our knowledge of the importance of hepatitis B in the pathogenesis of HCC has led to the trial of a viral vaccine in the hope of preventing a human cancer.

References

Ablashi DV, Easton JM, Guegar JH: Herpes viruses and cancer in man and subhuman primates. *Biomed* **24**:286–305, 1976.

Adam E, Kaufman RH, Adler-Storthz K, *et al:* A prospective study of association of herpes simplex virus and papilloma virus infection with cervical neoplasia in women exposed to diethylstilbesterol in utero. *Int J Cancer* **25**:3519–3526, 1985.

Bartholomew CF, Cleghorn C, Wavenau P, *et al:* HTLV-1 and tropical spastic paraparesis. *Lancet* **2**:99–100, 1986.

Beasley P: The major etiology of hepatocellular carcinoma, in Fortner JG, Rhoads JE (eds): *Accomplishments in Cancer Research.* Philadelphia, JP Lippincott, 1987, pp 80–106.

Beasley RP: Overview of the epidemiology of hepatocellular carcinoma. Presented at the 1990 International Symposium on Viral Hepatitis and Liver Disease, Houston, Texas, April 4–8, 1990.

Beasley P, Hwang L-Y, Lin C-C, *et al:* Hepatocellular carcinoma and hepatitis B virus. A prospective study of 22,707 men in Taiwan. *Lancet* **2**:1129–1132, 1981.

Beral V, Peterman T, Berkelman R, *et al:* AIDS-associated non-Hodgkin lymphoma. *Lancet* **337**:805–809, 1991.

Biggar RJ: Cancer in acquired immunodeficiency syndrome. An epidemiological assessment. *Sem Onc* **17**:251–260, 1990.

Biggar RJ, Rabkin CS: Lymphomas in the AIDS era. *Curr Op Oncol* (in press).

Birx DL, Redfield RR, Tosato G: Defective regulation of Epstein–Barr virus infection in acquired immunodeficiency syndrome (AIDS) or AIDS-related disorders. *N Engl J Med* **314**:874–879, 1986.

Blattner WA: Retroviruses, in Evans AS (ed): *Viral Infections of Humans: Epidemiology and Control,* 3rd ed. New York, Plenum Press, 1989, pp 545–592.

Boshart M, Gissman L, Ikenberg H, *et al:* A new type of papilloma virus DNA, its presence in genital cancer biopsies, and in cell lines derived from cervical cancer. *EMBO J* **3:**1151–1157, 1984.

Burkitt DP: A sarcoma involving the jaws in African children. *Br J Surg* **46:**218–223, 1958.

Burkitt DP: Determining the climatic limitations of a children's tumor in Africa. *Br Med J* **2:**1019–1023, 1962.

Chan KC, Mueller N, Evans A, *et al:* Epstein–Barr virus antibody patterns preceding the diagnosis of nasopharyngeal carcinoma. *Cancer Causes Control* **2:**125–131, 1991.

Deinhart F: Oncogenic herpes viruses in species other than owl monkeys. A review. *J Med Primatol* **3:**79–88, 1974.

de The G, Geser A, Day NE, *et al:* Epidemiological evidence for a causal relationship between Epstein–Barr virus and Burkitt's lymphoma from Ugandan prospective study. *Nature* **274:**756–761, 1978.

de The G, Ho JHC, Muir CS: Nasopharyngeal carcinoma, in Evans AS (ed): *Viral Infections of Humans: Epidemiology and Control,* 3rd ed. New York, Plenum Press, 1989, pp 737–787.

de Villiers EM, Wagner D, Schneider A, *et al:* Human papilloma infections in women with and without abnormal cervical cytology. *Lancet* **2:**703–706, 1987.

Doll R, Peto R: The causes of cancer: Quantitative estimates of avoidable risks in the United States today. *J Natl Cancer Inst* **66:**1196–1265, 1981.

Epstein MA, Achong BG, Barr YM: Virus particles in cultured lymphoblasts from Burkitt's lymphoma. *Lancet* **1:**702–703, 1964.

Epstein MA, Hunt RD, Rabin H: Pilot experiments with EB virus in owl monkeys (*Aotus trivirgatus*). 1. Reticuloproliferative disease in an inoculated animal. *Int J Cancer* **12:**309–318, 1973.

Essex M, Cotter SM, Stephenson JR, *et al: Leukemia, lymphoma, and fibrosarcoma of cats as models for similar diseases of man.* Cold Spring Harbor Lab, 1977, pp 1197–1214.

Evans AS: Viruses, in Schottenfeld D, Fraumeni J (eds): *Cancer Epidemiology and Prevention.* Philadelphia, W B Saunders Co, 1982, pp 364–390.

Evans AS: Epidemiology of Burkitt's lymphoma: Other risk factors, in: Lenoir GM, O'Connor GT, Olweny CLM (eds): *Burkitt's Lymphoma: A Human Cancer Model.* Lyons, IARC, 1985, pp 197–204.

Evans AS, Comstock GW: Presence of elevated antibody titers to Epstein–Barr virus before Hodgkin's disease. *Lancet* **1:**1183–1186, 1981.

Evans AS, de The G: Burkitt lymphoma, in Evans AS (ed): *Viral Infections of Humans: Epidemiology and Control,* 3rd ed. New York, Plenum Press, 1989, pp 713–735.

Evans AS, Mueller N: Viruses and cancer. Causal associations. *Ann Epidemiol* **1:**71–92, 1990.

Evans AS, Cox F, Nankervis G, *et al:* A health and serological survey of a community in Barbados. *Int J Epidemiol* **3:**167–175, 1974.

Ferell PB, Aitcheson CT, Pearson GR, *et al:* Seroepidemiological study of relationships between Epstein–Barr virus and rheumatoid arthritis. *J Clin Invest* **67:**681–687, 1981.

Gerin JL, Tennant BC, Ponzetto A, *et al:* The woodchuck animal model of hepatitis B-like virus infection and disease. *Prog Biol Res* **143:**23–38, 1983.

Geser A, de The G, Lenoir G, *et al:* Final case reporting from the Ugandan prospective study of the relationship between EBV and Burkitt's lymphoma. *Int J Cancer* **29:**397–400, 1982.

Granoff A: Lucke tumor-associated viruses—A review, in Biggs PM, de The G, Payne LN (eds): *Oncogenesis and Herpesviruses.* Lyons, France, IARC, 1972, pp 171–182.

Hamilton-Dutoit SJ, Pallesen G, Karkov J, *et al:* Identification of EBV-DNA in tumor cells of AIDS-related lymphoma by in situ hybridization. *Lancet* **1:**552–554, 1989.

Hadler SC, Margolis HS: Viral hepatitis, in Evans AS (ed): *Viral Infections of Humans: Epidemiology and Control,* 3rd ed. New York, Plenum Press, 1989, pp 351–391.

Hallee TJ, Evans AS, Niederman JC, *et al:* Infectious mononucleosis at the U.S. Military Academy. A prospective study in a single class over four years. *Yale Biol Med* **47:**182–195, 1974.

Hanto DW, Sakomoto K, *et al:* The Epstein–Barr virus in the pathogenesis of post-transplant lymphoproliferative disorders. *Surg* **90:**204–213, 1981.

Hanto DW, Sakomoto K, Purtillo DT, *et al:* The Epstein–Barr virus in the pathogenesis of post-transplant lymphoproliferative disorders. *Surgery* **90:**204–213, 1981.

Herbst H, Niedobitek G, Kneba M, *et al:* High incidence of Epstein–Barr virus genomes in Hodgkin's disease. *Am J Clin Pathol* **137:**13–18; 1990.

Herbst H, Tippleman G, Anagnostopoulos I, *et al:* Immunoglobulin and T-cell receptor gene rearrangements in Hodgkin's and K-1-positive angioplastic large cell lymphoma dissociation between phenotype and genotype. *Leuk Res* **91:**103–116, 1991.

Hinuma Y, Komoda H, Chosa T, *et al:* Antibodies to adult T-cell leukemia virus associated antigen (ATLA) in sera from patients with ATL and controls in Japan. A nationwide sero-epidemiologic study. *Int J Cancer* **29:** 631–635, 1982.

Ho HC, Kwan HC, Ng MH, *et al:* Serum IgA antibodies to Epstein–Barr capsid antigen preceding symptoms of nasopharyngeal carcinoma. *Lancet* **1:**436–437, 1978.

Ho M, Miller G, Atchinson W, *et al:* Epstein–Barr virus infections and DNA hybridization studies in post-transplant lymphomas and lymphoproliferative lesions: The role of primary infections. *J Infect Dis* **152:**876–886, 1985.

Hunsmann G, Schneider J, Schmidt J, *et al:* Detection of serum antibodies to adult T-cell leukemia virus in non-human primates and in people from Africa. *Int J Cancer* **32:**329–352, 1983.

Kiyosawsa K, Sodeyama T, Tamaka E, *et al:* The causal relationship between non-A, non-B hepatocellular carcinoma (HCC) after post-transfusion hepatitis and hepatitis C virus. The 1990 Symposium on Viral Hepatitis and Liver Disease, April 4–8, 1990, Houston, Texas, Abstract 632.

Levine PH, Blattner WA: The epidemiology of human virus-associated hematologic malignancies. *Leuk* **6:**54s–59s, 1992.

Lindemalm C, Biberfield P, Biorkholm M, *et al:* Epstein–Barr virus-associated antibody pattern in untreated non-Hodgkin's lymphoma patients. Relationship to clinical variables and lymphocyte functions. *Int J Canc* **32:**675–682, 1983.

List AF, Greer JP, Cousar JP, *et al:* Non-Hodgkin's lymphoma after treatment of Hodgkin's disease: Association with Epstein–Barr virus. *Ann Int Med* **105:**668–673, 1986.

Lucke, B: Carcinoma in the leopard frog: Its probable causation by a virus. *J Exp Med* **68:**457–468, 1938.

Maeda Y, Furukawa M, Takehara Y, *et al:* Prevalence of possible T-cell leukemia virus carriers among volunteer blood donors in Japan: A nationwide study. *Int J Cancer* **33:**717–720, 1984.

Melnick J: Hepatocellular carcinoma caused by hepatitis B virus, in Evans AS (ed): *Viral Infections of Humans: Epidemiology and Control,* 3rd ed. New York, Plenum Press, 1989, pp 769–780.

Melnick JL, Rawls WE, Adam E: Cervical cancer, in Evans AS (ed): *Viral Infections of Humans: Epidemiology and Control,* 3rd ed. New York, Plenum Press, 1989, pp 687–711.

Miller G: Oncogenicity of Epstein–Barr virus. *J Infect Dis* **130:**187–205, 1974.

McGrath I: Pathogenesis of African Burkitt's lymphoma. Presented at the Fifth International Symposium of Epstein–Barr Virus and Associated Diseases, Annency, France, Sept. 13–19, 1992.

Masucci G, Mellstedt H, Masucci MG, *et al:* Immunological characterization of Hodgkin and non-Hodgkin's lymphoma patients with high antibody titers against Epstein–Barr virus-associated antigens. *Canc Res* **44:**1288–1300, 1984.

Mueller N: Epidemiological studies assessing the role of the Epstein–Barr virus in Hodgkin's disease. *Yale J Biol Med* **60:**321–327, 1987.

Mueller N: The epidemiology of HTLV-1 infections. *Cancer Causes Control* **2:**37–52, 1991.

Mueller NE, Evans AS, Harris N, *et al:* Hodgkin's disease and Epstein–Barr virus. Evidence of altered antibody pattern prior to diagnosis. *N Engl J Med* **320:**689–695, 1989.

Mueller N, Mohar A, Evans A, *et al:* Epstein–Barr virus antibody patterns preceding the diagnosis of non-Hodgkin's lymphoma. *Int J Cancer* **49:**387–393, 1991.

Mueller N, Evans AS, London WT: Viruses, in Schottenfeld D, Fraumeni J Jr (eds): *Cancer Epidemiology and Prevention,* 2nd ed. Philadelphia, W B Saunders Co, in press.

Mueller N, Mohar A, Evans A, *et al:* Epstein-Barr virus antibody patterns preceding the diagnosis of non-Hodgkin's lymphoma. *Int J Cancer* **49:**387–393, 1991.

Nahmias AJ, Josey WF: Herpes simplex viruses 1 and 2, in Evans AS (ed): *Viral Infections of Humans: Epidemiology and Control,* 3rd ed. New York, Plenum Press, 1989, pp 393–417.

The New York Times: Growth gene is linked to many cancers. April 23, 1991, pp C1, C9.

Pater MM, Pater A: Human papillomavirus types 16 and 18 sequences in carcinoma cell lines of the cervix. *Virology* **145:**313–318, 1985.

Pater MM, Dunne J, Hogan G, *et al:* Human papillomavirus types 16 and 18 sequences in early cervical neoplasia. *Virology* **155:**13–18, 1986.

Payne LN: Pathogenesis of Marek's disease. A review, in Biggs PM, de The G, Payne LN (eds): *Oncogenesis and Herpes Viruses.* Lyon, France, IARC Sci Pub, 1972, pp 21–37.

Poiesz BJ, Ruscetti FW, Gazdar AF, *et al:* Detection and isolation of type-C retrovirus particles from fresh and cultured lymphocytes from patients with cutaneous T-cell lymphoma. *Proc Natl Acad Sci USA* **77:**7415–7419, 1980.

Purtillo DT, Bhawan J, Hutt LM, *et al:* Epstein–Barr virus infections in the X-linked recessive lymphoproliferative syndrome. *Lancet* **1:**798–800, 1978.

Rabkin CS, Biggar RJ, Horn JW: Increasing incidence of cancer associated with human immunodeficiency virus outbreak. *Int J Cancer* **12:**692–696, 1991.

Rawls WE, Bacchetti S, Graham FL: Relationship of herpes simplex viruses to human malignancies. *Curr Top Microbiol Immunol* **77:**71–87, 1977.

Reeves WC, Caussy D, Brinton LA, *et al:* Case–control study of human papillomaviruses and cervical cancer in Latin America. *Int J Cancer* **40:**450–454, 1987.

Reidel DA, Evans AS, Saxinger C, *et al:* A historical survey of human T-cell leukemia/lymphoma virus type 1 (HTLV-1) transmission in Barbados. *J Infect Dis* **159:**603–609, 1989.

Robert-Guroff M, Gallo RC: Establishment of an etiologic relationship between the human T-cell leukemia/lymphoma virus (HTLV) and adult T-cell leukemia. *Blut* **47:**1–12, 1983.

Rosenblatt JD, Chen ISY, Wachsman W: Infection with HTLV-1 and HTLV-2. Evolving concepts. *Semin Hematol* **25:**230–246, 1988.

Schneider-Gadecke A, Schwarz E: Different human cervical carcinoma cell lines show similar transcription of human papillomavirus type 18 early genes. *EMBO J* **55:**2285–2292, 1986.

Shope T, Dechairo D, Miller G: Malignant lymphoma in cotton-top marmosets following inoculation of Epstein–Barr virus. *Proc Natl Acad Sci USA* **70:**2487–2491, 1973.

Smotkin D, Wellstein FO: Transcription of human papillomavirus type 16 early genes in a cervical cancer and a cancer-derived cell line and identification of the E 7 protein. *Proc Natl Acad Sci USA* **83:**4680–4684, 1986.

Szmuness W: Hepatocellular carcinoma and hepatitis B virus: Evidence for a causal association. *Prog Med Virol* **2:**207–214, 1978.

Tajima K, and Hinumo Y: Epidemiological features of adult T-cell leukemia virus, in Mathe G, Reizenstein P (eds.): *Pathophysiological Aspects of Cancer.* Oxford, Pergamon Press, 1984, pp 75–85.

Uccini S, Monardo F, Stoppacciaro A, *et al:* High frequency of Epstein–Barr virus genome detection in Hodgkin's disease of HIV-positive patients. *Int J Cancer* **46:**581–585, 1990.

Vacini A, Mangari V, Stoppacciaro A, *et al:* High frequency of Epstein–Barr virus genome detection in Hodgkin's disease. *Int J Canc* **46:**581–585, 1990.

Vonka V, Kanka J, Jelinek J, *et al:* Prospective study on the relationship between cervical neoplasia and herpes simplex type-2 virus. I. Epidemiological characteristics. *Int J Cancer* **33:**49–60, 1984.

Weiss LM, Movahed LA, Warhke RK, *et al:* Detection of Epstein–Barr viral genomes in Reed–Sternberg cells of Hodgkin's disease. *N Engl J Med* **320:**502–506, 1989.

Weiss S: Unpublished data quoted by Blattner, 1989.

Yasumoto S, Burkhardt AL, Doniger J, *et al:* Human papillomavirus type 16 DNA-induced malignant transformation of NIH 3T3 cells. *J Virol* **57:**572–577, 1986.

Yoshida M, Hahari S, Seike M: Molecular biology of human T-cell leukemia virus, in *Microbiology and Immunology,* vol 5, No. 115. Berlin, Springer, 1985, pp 157–175.

Zeng Y, Zhang LG, Li HY, *et al:* Serological mass survey for early detection of nasopharyngeal carcinoma in Wu-Zhou City, China. *Int J Cancer* **29:**129–141, 1982.

Zeng Y, Zhang JM, Li LY, *et al:* Follow up studies on Epstein–Barr virus IgA/VCA antibody positive persons in Zwabgwu County, China. *Intervirology* **20:**190–194, 1983.

Zur Hausen H: Human papilloma viruses and their possible role in squamous cell carcinomas. *Curr Top Microbiol Immunol* **78:**1–30, 1977.

Zur Hausen H: Human genital cancer: Synergism between two virus infections and initiating events. *Lancet* **2:**1370–1372, 1982.

Zur Hausen H: Genital papillomavirus infections. *Prog Med Virol* **32:**15–21, 1985.

Zur Hausen H: Intracellular surveillance of persisting viral infections. Human genital cancer results from deficient cellular control of papillomavirus gene expression. *Lancet* **2:**489–491, 1986.

Zur Hausen H: Papillomaviruses in human cancer. *Cancer* **59:**1692–1696, 1987a.

Zur Hausen H: Papillomaviruses in human carcinogenesis. Presented at Symposium on Tumor Biology, The Karolinska Institute, Stockholm, August 20–21, 1987b.

Zur Hausen H, Papilloma/host cell interaction in the pathogenesis of anorectal cancer, in: *Origins of Human Cancer: A Comprehensive Review.* New York, Cold Spring Harbor Lab Press, 1991a, pp 685–688.

Zur Hausen H: Viruses in human cancers. *Science* **254:**1167–1173, 1991b.

6

Causation of Epidemics and Immunological Diseases

This chapter will review the evidence for causation in two contrasting disease groups. In the first, epidemic diseases, the proof of the means of transmission of the infectious agent goes back to the work of John Snow and the transmission of cholera; the proof of the microbiological cause of an epidemic became possible in the late 1800s, when methods for isolating bacteria became possible. The methods employed in epidemic investigation for seeking both the method of transmission and the proof of causation by a specific infectious agent have become quite standardized, particularly through the work of the Centers for Disease Control in the United States. The second disease group, that of immunological diseases, is one in which the criteria for establishing the nature of an immunological disease and for proof of the relationship of pathological changes to autoimmunization are of recent origin. In fact, there are few published guidelines on establishing causal relationships between exposure to a specific agent and most immune-mediated diseases.

For the sake of brevity, discussion of epidemic diseases and of immunological diseases have been combined into one chapter.

Epidemic Diseases

An important task of the public health epidemiologist is to establish the cause of an outbreak or epidemic so that appropriate methods for its control can be instituted. The methods employed in epidemic investigation are reviewed elsewhere (Evans, 1986, 1990, 1991; Frost, 1941; Fonseca and Armenian, 1991; Gregg, 1986; Stanley, 1977) and will not be discussed here. This chapter will discuss the proof of one of the steps in such investigation—the proof of the hypothesis of causation.

An epidemic can be defined as an increase in the number of cases of a disease or clinical syndrome as compared with the number of cases in the same time period and place in the past. Outbreaks may be of infectious, toxic, chemical, drug, psychological, or other noninfectious origin and the time period involved may be days, months, or years. Even the incubation period of infectious diseases may stretch over years; e.g., AIDS has an average incubation period of 11.5 years, and kuru, 27 years (Klitzman *et al.*, 1984). Over the long perspective, the rise and fall in the incidence of coronary artery disease and of lung cancer may be considered as consistent with the curve of epidemic diseases.

This chapter will propose a list of guidelines for establishing causal proof that a given agent is responsible for a specific outbreak, and then refer to some early and classical epidemics mentioned elsewhere in this book.

Table 6.1 presents possible elements of proof in implicating an agent in an outbreak of infectious disease.

A number of epidemics or outbreaks are discussed elsewhere in this book. These include mention of epidemics in the prebacteriological era such as scurvy, lead colic, the cholera outbreaks in London in 1849 and 1854, and puerperal

Table 6.1
Guidelines for Establishing Causation in an Infectious Disease Epidemic

1. The agent should be isolated from the majority of cases involved in the epidemic.
2. The agent should be isolated more commonly in sick than in well persons (but a high incidence of subclinical infections may obscure this difference).
3. The incubation period of the agent isolated should correspond to that of the disease.
4. Antibody to the agent should appear during illness, or a fourfold or greater rise in titer should occur, or an agent-specific IgM antibody should be demonstrated.
5. Intervention measures that abolish the source of exposure to the agent, or interrupt its means of transmission, or which protect the host by agent-specific active or passive immunization should control the epidemic. Treatment or prophylaxis with an antibiotic or antiviral agent to which the organism is sensitive that halts epidemic spread is indirect evidence of a causal association but is usually not agent-specific.
6. Reproduction of the disease in susceptible experimental animals with evidence of spread by a similar route of transmission.
7. No other agent should show the same causal associations, unless it is the rare instance in which two infectious agents are needed to produce the clinical picture. (HIV and the opportunistic infections of AIDS is an example.)

sepsis, all of which are discussed in Chapter 1. More recent outbreaks of bacterial disease, such as Legionnaire's disease and Lyme disease, are presented in Chapter 2, and that of AIDS, associated with the human immunodeficiency virus (HIV or HTLV-III), is reviewed in Chapter 3, along with the controversy involved in the causal relation of the virus to the clinical manifestations of the disease.

Immunological Diseases

The immune system is a key component in our defenses against many diseases, especially infectious diseases. In this process, both the affected as well as normal tissues may be damaged. In addition, the interactions between the humoral arm—performed primarily through B cells—and the cell-mediated arm—whose activities are carried out primarily through a variety of T lymphocytes and macrophages—are complex and are subject to immunoregulatory mechanisms which may go awry. The abnormalities occurring in normal immune function may result from genetic defects, from acquired diseases, or from drug-induced immunodeficiencies as in renal transplant recipients. This section will discuss the definition of what constitutes an immunological disease and the evidence needed to establish proof of causation for a specific antigen. In addition to diseases that are primarily immunological in nature, the immune system also plays an important role in the mechanisms in which damage is caused by infectious agents, especially viruses. These have been well reviewed by Notkins and associates (Notkins and Koproski, 1973; Notkins, 1974; Notkins and Oldstone, 1984; and Mims (1982). The same immune processes that control infectious diseases may sometimes result in damage to normal tissues. These immune mechanisms include: (1) Antibody produced by the infectious agent may circulate until it encounters the antigen and in combining with it may initiate damage to the tissue that is infected, or to which the agent is attached. (2) Immune complexes may form between the antigen and the antibody produced to it; when these complexes represent a balance between the two components or with a slight antigen excess, then combination with complement occurs and they are deposited in blood vessels, especially those in the glomeruli of the kidney, producing an inflammatory reaction and tissue injury in combination with polymorphonuclear cells, which is manifested as an immune complex nephritis. Some infectious agents, especially viruses, induce new antigenic properties on the surface membranes of infected cells which may be regarded as foreign by the host's T lymphocytes. These then react in antibody and cell-mediated responses, leading to tissue injury or immune complexes. An example of this is the neoantigen induced by Epstein–Barr virus (EBV) on the B lymphocytes it infects. T lymphocytes then respond to this neoantigen by transformation and proliferation, and a mixed B–T lymphocyte interaction results. Functional changes, consisting of alterations in the production, characteristics, or release of cellular products may also occur without inducing cell damage *per se* (Notkins and Oldstone, 1984).

This chapter will not deal with these B- and T-cell reactions during infection because they are concerned with the *mechanisms* involved in tissue injury, not the causal relationship of the infectious agent to disease itself. Instead, attention will be directed to (1) the criteria establishing the immunological nature of a disease, (2) the criteria for proof of the relation of pathological changes to autoimmuniza-tion, and (3) modifications in the Koch postulates for immune-mediated disease. While the criteria overlap considerably, they have been formulated by different immunologists, each with a particular view of the subject. I have been able to find only a few such criteria published in the literature for immunological dis-eases, so I will reproduce them verbatim. I feel incompetent in the field to synthesize the various criteria into a general one. The interactions are so com-plex, often involving a cascade of interdependent events, that it is difficult to separate them into initiating (causal) and promoting events and those that are cofactors.

Immunological Nature of a Disease

The criteria for an immunological disease have been defined by Dr. Byron Waksman (Figure 6.1), an eminent American immunologist, and formerly Chair-man of Microbiology and Immunology at Yale University (Waksman, 1962). They are reproduced in Table 6.2. The first two criteria resemble those for an infectious agent in that there is a definitive agent that initiates the "immunizing event" in the same fashion that a virus or bacterium initiates an infection. Then,

Table 6.2
Criteria for Immunological Nature of a Disease[a]

---

1. A well-defined *immunizing event* followed by a *latent period* preceding appearance of hypersensitive state.
2. *Shortened* latent period after secondary stimulation.
3. *Passive transfer* of immune state to normal recipients with serum or "sensitized" cells.
4. *Suppression* of the immune state by administration of the antigen in proper manner by desensitization or by tolerance.

These criteria must show specificity, i.e., the same or very similar antigens needed to invoke each of the phenomena.

---

[a]Derived from Waksman (1962).

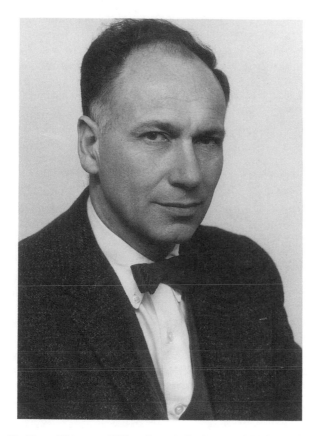

Figure 6.1. Dr. Byron Waksman, 1919– , formerly Professor and Chairman, Department of Microbiology, Yale University School of Medicine.

as in an infectious disease, there is a latent or incubation period before the clinical manifestations occur. In immunological diseases, a shortened latent period to disease manifestations occurs when reexposed to the same or similar immunogen, whereas in most infectious diseases, immunity usually results after first exposure to the antigen and protects against either infection or disease resulting from reexposure. However, the time period from this reexposure to an increase in antibody production is shorter than that after the first exposure and is termed an anamnestic response, or booster effect.

There are also exceptions to the concept that high protection and immunity results from exposure to all infectious agents. Examples in which immunity is ineffective, or only partially protective, include susceptibility to repeated attacks of gonorrhea, or repeated reinfections with respiratory syncytial virus, or the reinfection or endogenous reactivation that is characteristic of many herpesviruses, such as herpes simplex or cytomegalovirus. Recent evidence indicates that certain viruses can coexist in the presence of antibody and the person remain infectious to others. Examples of this are HIV, human T-cell leukemia/lymphoma virus (HTLV-I), and hepatitis C virus (HCV).

As to the third criterion, dealing with the transfer of the immune state to other hosts by the transfer of serum or "sensitized" cells, this effect is in contrast to that in infectious diseases in which protection, not susceptibility, is transferred in this manner. Thus, the passive transfer of serum from persons convalescent from an infectious disease, or of gamma globulins prepared therefrom, usually confers protection against infection with that agent, albeit of a temporary nature. This concept is the basis for the prevention of several viral infections, such as rubella and hepatitis A. In contrast, in immunological diseases, such transfer of serum or sensitized T lymphocytes carries with it to the recipient susceptibility to disease when exposure to that immunogen occurs again. Examples are serum sickness and experimental allergic encephalitis. The latter is an example of the transfer of sensitized cells as published by Dr. Waksman (Waksman, 1959) and Patterson (1966).

The fourth criterion, suppression of the immune state by proper dosages of the antigen, is a unique immunological process for protection against reactions following subsequent exposures to the immunizing agent. It is unlike that of an infectious disease in which the antigen is administered, as in a vaccine, to protect against the consequences of primary exposure to the antigen.

The high degree of specificity for the antigen in the production of immunological diseases is also dissimilar to infectious diseases in which a variety of different antigens are capable of inducing a similar clinical syndrome, as exemplified by the multiple microbiological forms capable of resulting in similar clinical syndromes involving the respiratory tract, or the gastrointestinal system, or the central nervous system.

Relation of Pathological Changes to Autoimmunization

The diseases associated with autoimmunity are being increasingly recognized and investigated. The late Dr. Ernst Witebsky (Figure 6.2) was an important early investigator in the analysis of these diseases, especially in his work on autoimmune diseases of the thyroid gland. He was Chairman of the Department of Microbiology at the University of Buffalo. His criteria for proof of a causative relationship of pathological changes to autoimmunization are shown in Table 6.3. In many ways they resemble the Henle–Koch postulates in that they require the demonstration of the causal factor, here cell-bound antibodies, the characterization, and even isolation, of the antigen that produced them, and the experimental reproduction of the antibodies (but not necessarily the disease) in experi-

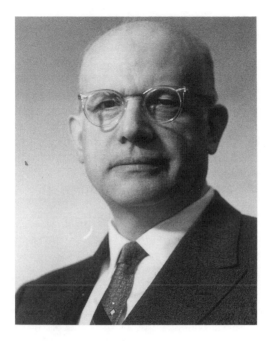

Figure 6.2. Ernst Witebsky, M.D., 1901–1969, Professor and Chairman, Department of Microbiology, University of Buffalo School of Medicine.

mental animals. Other diseases based on an immunological component that may have been induced by a virus are systemic lupus erythematosis, juvenile diabetes, sarcoidosis, rheumatoid arthritis, polyarteritis nodosa, Sjogren's syndrome, and certain diseases of the central nervous system in which antimyelin protein immune responses are involved, or in which disturbances in amyloid occur. In some, the immune disturbance results from a genetic disturbance, such as recent evidence of a gene regulating amyloid activity in Alzheimer's disease.

Table 6.3
Criteria for Proof of Relation of Pathological Changes to Autoimmunization[a]

1. Demonstration in the serum of cell-bound antibodies.
2. The antigen against which the antibody is directed should be characterized or even isolated.
3. Antibodies should be produced against the same antigen in experimental animals.

[a]From Witebsky (1959).

Table 6.4
Updated Koch's Postulates for Immune-Mediated Disease[a]

1. The immunoreactants should be demonstrable in every case of the disease.
2. The immunoreactants should be able to demonstrate *in vitro* an activity associated with disease pathogenesis.
3. Upon transfer to a normal individual, the immunoreactant should be able to confer the disease.

[a]From P. W. Askenase (personal communication, February 8, 1989).

Criteria for Immune-Mediated Disease

I am indebted to my colleague, Dr. Philip W. Askenase, Professor of Medicine and Pathology and Chief, Section of Allergy and Clinical Immunology at Yale University, for the criteria listed in Table 6.4, as well as for the example of its application. His criteria contain some of the concepts of those of Waksman and of Witebsky, but are presented in a format of updated Koch's postulates for immune-mediated diseases. His best example for these postulates is that of antibodies to the acetylcholine receptor in the autoimmune disease called myasthenia gravis. He states: "Firstly, in this disease, all of the patients (and all of the animals with the experimental model of the disease) have antibodies and/or sensitized cells reactive with acetylcholine receptors of the neuromuscular junction. Secondly, *in vitro* these antibodies can induce the miniature end plate potential abnormalities that are electrophysiologically characteristic of this disease. Finally, these antibodies on transfer to normal individuals produce neuromuscular weakness that can be overcome by acetylcholine esterase drug treatment (i.e., transfer of human immunoglobulins to mice or transfer of maternal IgG to neonates resulting in clinical neonatal myasthenia)." Dr. Askenase emphasizes that this example is a rare one that proves the rule (i.e., the criteria for causation), but despite its rarity is an ideal worth pursuing in other instances.

References

Evans AS: Epidemic investigation, in Kelsey J, Thompson WW, Evans AS (eds): *Methods in Observational Epidemiology.* London, Oxford University Press, 1986, pp 212–253.
Evans AS: Epidemiological concepts, in Evans AS (ed): *Viral Infections of Humans: Epidemiology and Control,* 3rd ed. New York, Plenum Press, 1990, pp 3–49.

Evans AS: Introduction and concepts, in: *Bacterial Infections of Humans: Epidemiology and Control,* 2nd ed. New York, Plenum Press, 1991, pp 3–57.

Fonseca MGP, Armenian HK: Use of the case–control method in epidemic investigation. *Am J Epidemiol* **133:**748–752, 1991.

Frost WH: Epidemiology, in Macy KF (ed): *Papers of Wade Hampton Frost, M.D.* New York, The Commonwealth Fund, 1941.

Gregg MB: The principles of epidemic investigation, in: Chappie A, Holland WW, Detels R, *et al* (eds): *Oxford Textbook of Public Health.* London, Oxford University Press, 1986, vol 3, pp 284–297.

Klitzman RL, Alpers MP, Gajdusek DC: The natural incubation period of kuru and the episodes of transmission in three clusters of patients. *Neuroepidemiol* **3:**3–20, 1984.

Mims CA: *Pathogenesis of Infectious Diseases,* 2nd ed. New York, Academic Press, 1982.

Notkins AL: Commentary: Immune mechanism by which the spread of viral infections is stopped. *Cell Immunol* **11:**478–483, 1974.

Notkins AL: Molecular biology and viral pathogenesis. *N Engl J Med* **312:**507–509, 1985.

Notkins AL, Koproski N: How the immune response to a virus can cause disease. *Sci Am* **226:**22–31, 1973.

Notkins AL, Oldstone BA: *Concepts on Viral Pathogenesis.* Berlin, Springer-Verlag, 1984.

Patterson PY: Experimental allergic encephalomyelitis and autoimmune disease. *Adv Immunol* **5:**131–208, 1966.

Stanley JS: Investigation of disease outbreaks: Principles of epidemiology. Atlanta, Centers for Disease Control, 1977. (Home study course 3030-G.)

Waksman B: Allergic encephalomyelitis in rats and rabbits pretreated with nervous tissue. *J Neuropathol Exp Neurol* **18:**397–417, 1959.

Waksman B: Autoimmunity. *Medicine* **41:**92–141, 1962.

Witebsky E: Historical roots of present concepts of immunopathology, in *Immunogy-Immunologie 1st Int Symp, 1958.* Basel/Stuttgart, Benno Schabe & Co, Verlag, 1959, pp 1–19.

Limitations of the Henle–Koch Postulates

*Effect of New Concepts and of Technology**

Robert Koch early recognized that the postulates of causation he had included in 1882 in papers on the etiology of tuberculosis (Koch, 1882a,b; 1938) had their limitations. In a subsequent paper on bacteriological research presented at the International Medical Congress in Berlin (see Koch, 1890) he stated that while the bacteria of anthrax, tuberculosis, tetanus, and many animal diseases fully fulfilled his postulates, many others did not. These latter included the organisms of typhoid fever, diphtheria, leprosy, relapsing fever, and Asiatic cholera. The biggest problem was the failure to reproduce "the disease anew" in an experimental animal. He therefore felt that fulfillment of only the first two postulates was necessary to establish causation. Many other diseases have subsequently failed to fulfill the three postulates, or even two of them. In this chapter, I will discuss the limitations of the postulates from three standpoints: (1) those limitations that directly affected each of the three postulates, as stated in Rivers's (1937) translation, (2) the effect of newer concepts of pathogenesis and epidemiology on the need to modify the postulates, and (3) the influence of new technological developments that permitted identification of new organisms that could not be grown in pure culture, even if one includes tissue cultures for viruses as the equivalent of standard culture methods for bacteria. A summary of the limitations of the postulates is given in Table 7.1 as derived from previous publications (Evans 1977, 1980).

---

*A modified version of this article has appeared in the Yale Journal of Biological Medicine (Evans, 1991b).

Table 7.1
Limitations of Koch's[a] Postulates of Causation

1. Not applicable to all pathogenic bacteria
2. May not be applicable to viruses, fungi, parasites
3. Do not include the following concepts:
   - A. The asymptomatic carrier state
   - B. The biological spectrum of disease
   - C. Epidemiological elements of causation
   - D. Immunological elements of causation
   - E. Prevention of disease by elimination of putative cause as element of causation
   - F. Multiple causation
   - G. One syndrome has different causes in different settings
   - H. Reactivation of latent agents can cause disease
   - I. Immunological processes as cause of diseases

[a]More properly termed the Henle–Koch postulates.

Factors Directly Limiting the Henle–Koch Postulates as Originally Stated

"Postulate 1: (a) The parasite occurs in every case of the disease in question, and (b) under circumstances which can account for the pathological changes and clinical course of the disease." The first part of this postulate suggests that the organism is always *demonstrable* in every case of the disease, a situation that may not always be possible to establish if the organism is a difficult one to culture or if its occurrence preceded the development of the clinical signs, so that an appropriate specimen cannot be obtained. This happens if the clinical manifestations appear at the time when, or shortly after, antibody develops, which combines with the agent making its isolation difficult. This often occurs in viral infections, such as poliomyelitis and infectious mononucleosis.

In the second part of the first postulate, the need to demonstrate that the circumstances under which the organism is isolated "can account for the pathological changes and clinical course of the disease" is satisfied by those organisms in which tissue injury is the direct result of the inflammatory changes induced at the site of multiplication. This is true of many bacterial infections, and is applicable to the tissue damage due to direct lysis of tissues by many viruses. However, there are many exceptions to this concept. The production of disease by bacterial toxins that exert their effect at a site distant from the point of multiplication is an example of this problem. There are three common diseases in which this occurs.

(1) In diphtheria, the organisms multiply locally on epithelial surfaces, where they produce a powerful toxin, which spreads by the blood to the heart and nervous system, resulting in serious involvement in these distant sites. (2) Tetanus bacillus (*Clostridium tetani*) grows in infected wounds, or through a contaminated splinter, or in the umbilical cord of the newborn, where it produces a protein toxin that travels along the axons of peripheral nerves, reaching motor neurons, and eventually diffusing through the central nervous system. There, it binds to a ganglioside receptor, and similar to strychnine, interferes with anterior horn cell activity. (3) The third example is that of scarlet fever in which an erythrogenic strain of streptococcus (*Streptococcus pyogenes*) elaborates a toxin when it is itself infected with a temperate bacteriophage; the toxin then spreads from the local site of bacterial multiplication to the skin via the blood, resulting in the rash that is characteristic of scarlet fever.

Another unusual situation is that in cholera where, despite the enormous outpouring of fluid from the intestinal mucosa which leads to severe dehydration and sometimes death, *no* pathological changes in the involved intestine have been seen pathologically on intestinal biopsy (Gangarosa *et al.,* 1960). The outpouring of fluid is due to a complicated series of chemical events induced by an exotoxin and by a neuraminidase (or sialidase) produced by the organism.

Other indirect mechanisms of tissue injury not explicable simply by the mere presence of the organism involve immunological events. One example is the formation of immune complexes of antigen and antibody of a critical size, such as occurs in the glomerulonephritis that follows infections by certain strains of streptococcus, in the nephrotic syndrome that occurs in severe malarial infections, and in the secondary stage of syphilis. Similarly, the occurrence of rheumatic fever in the wake of group A hemolytic streptococcal infections involves a poorly understood immunological mechanism, perhaps related to the production of an antibody due to an antigen shared by the organism and by heart muscle. In viral infections, a wide variety of immunological responses may lead to the clinical manifestations of the disease. These have been classified as anaphylactic, cytotoxic, immune complex, and cell-mediated, and are discussed in Chapters 3 and 4. They are simply mentioned here to indicate that the establishment of the circumstances under which an organism can account for the pathological changes and clinical course of a disease is sometimes much more difficult than suggested by the Henle–Koch postulates. While the relationship between the organism and the disease should make general biological sense, knowledge of the exact pathogenic events leading to tissue damage often comes long after the organism has been fully accepted as the cause of the disease.

"Postulate 2: It occurs in no other disease as a fortuitous and nonpathogenic parasite." This implies that the organism should always display pathogenicity and not exist as "an accidental tourist" in the presence of some other disease. Several limitations to this concept arose almost immediately. The first was the discovery that organisms could persist long after recovery from the clinical disease. Thus, an organism, say organism A, could still be present and isolable when the individual developed a subsequent disease due to organism B. A second circumstance was when organism A resulted in a completely asymptomatic, subclinical infection and at the same time the patient was infected with organism B, which was the real culprit in producing the clinical manifestations. The third circumstance is when organism A exists in a completely latent state until organism B infects the individual producing an illness, but also reactivating organism A from latency to active, asymptomatic multiplication. Many bacterial forms, especially intracellular organisms, such as the tubercle bacillus, brucella, parasitic infections like malaria, and many viruses, especially of the herpes family, are examples of these three possible circumstances.

Historically, the discovery of the asymptomatic and carrier state occurred shortly after Koch's 1890 lecture in Berlin. In 1893, Koch, himself, demonstrated the existence of a convalescent carrier state for the cholera bacillus, as well as the presence of a healthy carrier state, although he did not place much emphasis at that time on the latter in the transmission of the infection (Koch, 1893). At the same time, Park and Beebe in the United States clearly established both the importance of the carrier state in diphtheria and the importance of the healthy carrier in its transmission within a family (Park and Beebe, 1894). In a third disease, typhoid fever, the role of the healthy carrier in the spread of infection was recognized by Reed *et al.* (1900) in studies of the disease in military camps during the Spanish–American war in 1898 and later by Koch (1903). The importance of the long-term carrier state of the typhoid bacillus was later illustrated by the famous case of Mary Mallon, known as "Typhoid Mary," whose chronic carrier state and occupation as a household cook resulted in a series of outbreaks in New York City over almost two decades, as described by Soper (1907, 1939). The carrier state has been reviewed by Ledingham and Arkwright (1912).

Had Koch known in 1882 of the asymptomatic and carrier states and of the persistence of the organism long after recovery, it is not clear how they would have affected his phrasing of the second postulate. His concern was in establishing the *pathogenicity* of the tubercle bacillus, not its *nonpathogenicity,* and to stress that its isolation from cases was a constant feature, not the accidental growth of some nonpathogenic, contaminating organism that had nothing to do with the disease in question. This same issue has plagued microbiologists ever since, both in differentiating the pathogenicity of two or more organisms isolated from involved tissues of an ill person, as well as the presence in experimental animals or tissue cultures of indigenous organisms derived from the animal or tissue itself, or from airborne, commensal organisms contaminating the culture media. Today, we would insist that the presence of such extraneous organisms be fully excluded by careful studies of uninoculated animals or media and/or confirmation of the results in several laboratories.

"Postulate 3: (a) After being fully isolated from the body and repeatedly grown in pure culture, (b) it can induce the disease anew." The growth in pure, or even impure culture is not possible for many bacteria. Let me give two examples. The leprosy bacillus, *Mycobacterium leprae,* was discovered by Hansen in 1874 (Hansen, 1875), and known as a disease for some 2000 years, but has yet to be cultivated on artificial media or in tissue culture. It does multiply readily in the armadillo, but without reproducing the disease. Thus, it fails to meet both parts of the third postulate. *Chlamydia trachomatis,* the cause of trachoma, which was described in the Ebers papyrus papers in 1500 B.C. and causes a wide spectrum of other clinical syndromes involving the eye, lung, and genital tract, cannot be cultivated on artificial media. However, it can be grown in the yolk sac of eggs and, much more easily, in certain types of tissue culture, such as McCoy cells, but even here requires centrifugation onto the medium to ensure growth (excepting the LGV strain). This organism, too, does not reproduce disease in an experimental animal. The limitations of the Henle–Koch postulates to viruses have been discussed in Chapters 3 and 4 but a couple of examples are of interest to reemphasize here. Hepatitis B virus cannot be grown in any type of tissue culture and fails to reproduce clinical hepatitis in experimental animals, although it multiplies in marmosets and chimpanzees. Thus, it fails to meet the two parts of the third postulate. Yet, an excellent vaccine has been prepared using virus circulating in infected humans as the source of antigen, and more recently, by DNA recombinant technology, in which the infectious nucleic acid is inserted into a yeast carrier. Hepatitis A virus has recently been grown in specialized tissue cultures after almost 40 years of failure to do so. From this successful propagation of the virus, efforts to produce both live and killed vaccines are under vigorous development, and at the moment a killed, attenuated vaccine has shown the most promise in vaccine trials. Rapid advances are occurring in identifying forms of viral hepatitis that are neither HAV nor HBV and were formerly designated in the past simply as "non-A, non-B" hepatitis, or NANB. One of these, which was transmitted by parenteral routes, and most closely resembled HBV in its epidemiology, has now been designated as type C (HCV). It produces severe and chronic forms of hepatitis that lead to cirrhosis, is the most common form of posttransfusion hepatitis in the developed world, where HBV has been controlled by screening blood donors, and is probably the major cause of hepatocellular carcinoma (HCC) not due to HBV. In Japan, for example, an increasing percentage of HCC is associated with HCV rather than HBV. The virus has been cloned, serological tests developed, and viral identification made by a nested polymerase chain reaction test in blood and tissues. A second type of non-A, non-B hepatitis has been identified that is transmitted by the fecal–oral route and is similar to hepatitis A (HAV), except that it produces high attack rates among adults and a high case–fatality rate in pregnant women. It has now been redesignated type E (for enteric) hepatitis (HEV). Its capacity to result in waterborne outbreaks has been deduced from earlier, large waterborne outbreaks, such as the one in India in the mid-1950s, by the lack of serological evidence of HAV infection. Diagnosis can now be made by immunoelectron microscopy on viral preparations from the stool. Neither HCV nor HEV has been grown in tissue culture, but both produce an asymptomatic infection of nonhuman primates, such as cynomolgous macaques, tamarins, and marmosets. Both viruses have been cloned so that rapid progress in diagnosis and vaccine developments may be expected. However, at the present time neither fulfill the Henle–Koch postulates.

In summary, many bacteria and viruses fail to fulfill the classical postulates of causation proposed by Henle and Koch, yet the agents are widely accepted as the cause of the diseases with which they are associated. Such incomplete evidence has not hampered successful efforts directed at their prevention and control. More modern criteria of causal proof should be used to establish causal inferences (Evans, 1976, 1988, 1991a).

Role of New Developments in Technology on Causation

Introduction

Our knowledge of the causation of infectious diseases depends on two major aspects: the conceptual and the technical. The former is concerned with our knowledge of the natural history of disease and its pathogenesis; the latter is concerned with the laboratory techniques available at the time to identify the organism, visualize it, grow it in the laboratory, reproduce the disease in an experimental animal, and explain how the organism causes the disease. The famous Henle–Koch postulates of causation (Table 2.5) (Henle, 1938; Koch, 1882a; 1938), which for over 100 years have guided investigators in establishing the causal relationship of an organism to a disease, were limited by conceptual issues, which have been reviewed (see Evans, 1976) and which have been summarized in Table 7.1.

This section will review the technical developments that preceded Koch and that permitted him to evolve his evidence of causation, particularly for tuberculosis. I will then present subsequent technical advances up to the present time that have permitted the identification of new organisms, each of which involved establishing the possible causal relationship to the disease from which it was isolated. In some cases, the discovery of the organism preceded recognition of the disease state with which it was associated. In other cases, the organism discovered by the new technique could not be cultivated in the laboratory or could not be reproduced in an experimental animal, thus not fulfilling the Henle–Koch postulates for causation.

Bacteriology

The major discoveries and examples of the organisms found are given in Table 7.2.

A few points should be emphasized at the start of this discussion. As has been stated so well by Bulloch (1938) in his great and comprehensive book, *The History of Bacteriology,* most advances have evolved in a series of small steps based on the work of several successive investigators, and the application of the method was not always made by its discoverer or even by those who later perfected the technique.

The discussion that follows was derived largely from the works of Bulloch (1938) and Foster (1970) for bacteriology and Fenner and Gibbs (1988) and Hughes (1977) for virology and in which the original references are cited. Bul-

Table 7.2
Technical Developments and the Discovery of Microbial Causes of Disease

Development	Examples
Light microscope	*Mycobacterium leprae*
Laboratory animals	
Guinea pigs	*M. tuberculosis,* Legionnaire's disease
Ferrets	Influenza
Adult mice	Herpes simplex, yellow fever
Suckling mice	Coxsackie, newer arboviruses
Chimpanzees	Hepatitis B, kuru, Creutzfeldt–Jakob
Armadillos	Leprosy
Bacterial culture (agar culture)	Most bacteria, especially Legionnaire's, campylobacteria, *Yersinia*
Embryonated eggs	Herpes, smallpox, some influenza viruses
Tissue culture	
Monkey kidney	Enteroviruses, Lassa
Adult human	Polio, adeno, RSV
Embryonic human	
Lung WI-38	CMV, rhinoviruses, corona virus
Cord lymphocytes	EBV, HIV, HTLV-I, HHV-6
Brain	Papova (JC strain)
Electron microscope	Hepatitis A, rotavirus, EVB
Fluorescent antibody	*M. pneumonia*, etiology of infectious mononucleosis

loch, in particular, has an excellent reference section and a brief sketch of all of the important microbiologists.

The Light Microscope

This instrument evolved at the end of the 16th or the beginning of the 17th century, and was based on much older knowledge of the art of making convex and concave lenses. The Dutch microscopist Antonie van Leeuwenhoek was said to have been the first to apply the light microscope to the identification of living protozoa and to bacteria (both in 1675) (Bulloch, 1938). This remarkable man ground his own lenses and made some 400 single biconvex microscopes (really more like magnifying glasses) that were capable of enlarging objects some 300 times. Besides his activities as a lens grinder and microscopist, he was also a draper, haberdasher, wine gauger for the town of Delft, and a qualified surveyor. His discoveries with his microscopes included descriptions of bacteria found in his own teeth and various morphological forms of bacteria such as coccal and spiral. His description of a motile animalcule that he found in his own feces was, in all probability, *Giardia lamblia,* and if so, it was the first parasitic protozoan to be observed in man (Dobell, 1932).

Bacterial Stains

Proper morphological description of organisms under the light microscope required some method of staining them to identify their characteristics better. The earliest efforts were apparently those of Hermann Hoffman in 1869 who employed carmine and fuchsin stains; the former was also used by Weigert in 1871 (Bulloch, 1938). However, the staining of bacteria as an art is said to have begun when Weigert showed that methyl violet stain can reveal cocci in tissues (Bulloch, 1938). Robert Koch improved on the method by preparing thin films on cover glasses, drying and fixing them in alcohol, and then using various stains, of which methyl violet 5B, fuchsin, and aniline brown were the most successful. Paul Ehrlich introduced methylene blue, and by adding an alkali to the dye, which allowed it to penetrate bacilli, Koch was able to identify the tubercle bacillus in 1882. This technique was also the basis of Löffler's methylene blue stain in 1884 (Löffler, 1884). Ehrlich improved the method of staining the tubercle bacillus by heating the slide and using aniline dye in a technique that was named the Ziehl–Nielsen acid-fast stain. Based on these observations, in 1884 Christian Gram, a Dane, developed (some say by accident) the stain that bears his name. This was made by adding Lugol's solution of iodine, followed by alcohol, and the Ehrlich stain (aniline–water–gentian violet). This stain is still used routinely today: every laboratory applies it to identify an unknown organism. Indeed, the first question in bacteriological classification is whether an organism is Gram-positive or Gram-negative.

Pure Cultures of Bacteria

In order to study specific bacteria, it was necessary to find both an appropriate medium for their pure culture and a technique to separate out individual organisms or clones to determine the homogeneity of the bacteria. Many workers were involved in these tasks, including Pasteur, Cohn, Löffler, and Klebs. Edwin Klebs (1834-1913) had worked with the tubercle bacillus and with anthrax at the same time as Koch, or even slightly before, and apparently made the first attempts to obtain separate cultures by a technique he termed "fractional method." Oscar Brefeld, a great mycologist, laid down the basic principles of obtaining pure cultures based on studies of fungi. These observations were published in 18 volumes. Joseph Lister, the Scottish surgeon who introduced aseptic techniques into the operating room, invented a specially constructed syringe with a graduated nut that could deliver volumes as small as 1/100 of a minum. After a millionfold dilution, he was able to deliver a drop containing a single bacterium. In this way he separated single colonies of *Bacterium lactis* in 1878. Other workers such as Nagele, Fitz, Hansen, and Salomonsen also used this dilution technique to obtain pure cultures. Parenthetically, it was this dilution technique by which Albert Sabin, some 100 years later, was able to obtain attenuated strains of poliomyelitis viruses that formed the basis of his oral vaccine. In bacterial cultures, it was Robert Koch who devised methods of isolating pure cultures that are still used today. His method was based on the use of clear nutrient gelatin with 1% meat extract. He prepared sterile slides, over which the medium was poured, inoculated with a platinum wire or needle, and then placed in a test tube with the sterile gelatin on a slant or upright. This method was demonstrated in 1881 with great acclaim before a very distinguished audience in London that included Lister and Pasteur. By 1883 Koch had improved the technique by mixing the bacterial inoculum with melted gelatin and pouring it over cold sterile glass plates. Students from all over the world flocked to Koch's laboratory in Berlin to learn the method. The ability to separate out and grow a single organism lent great specificity to the search for the causative agent of a disease. In virology, molecular techniques now permit identification of specific viruses, their genetic variability in human passage, and the genomic properties that determine pathogenicity and clinical response patterns. Epidemiologically, these tools in both bacteriology and virology have permitted tracing of epidemics due to a specific strain of the organism, to differentiate between reactivation of an agent and exogenous reinfection, and to identify many molecular characteristics of the microbial agent responsible for pathogenicity, virulence, and the pattern of host response. For example, a change in even one amino acid may alter a virus so that it is pathogenic, as is the case of rabies virus.

Virology

The technical developments discussed above for bacteriology had little impact on the field of virology because viruses differ from bacteria in at least two essential ways: (1) except for the large vaccinia virus, most viruses are smaller than bacteria and cannot be seen under the light microscope, which permits identification of bacteria; viruses thus require an electron microscope for their visualization. (2) Viruses cannot be grown in bacterial media but depend on living tissues for their multiplication, either in a living organism or in tissue cultures derived from human or animal tissues. Thus, the major developments that permitted virology to emerge as a separate discipline were based on filtration methods, by which viruses could be separated from bacteria and other large parasites, the discovery of the electron microscope, and the development of susceptible animal models and of tissue cultures.

The poxviruses represent the prototype virus type and smallpox the prototype disease on which most major developments in virology were first made. The large size of the virus, its ease of cultivation in the laboratory, and the characteristic features and epidemic importance of the disease it produced were the major reasons for this. The historical importance of the virus becomes very apparent when one reads Frank Fenner's chapter on "The Poxvirus" in the book *Portraits of Viruses,* which was edited by him and Adrian Gibbs (1988). The story of the conquest of smallpox has also been told in magnificent detail in a beautifully illustrated book, *Smallpox,* edited by Fenner, D. A. Henderson, and others (1989).

Viral Filters

In 1892, Dimitri Isoifirch Iwanowski, a graduate student at the University of St. Petersburg, discovered that tobacco mosaic virus could pass through a filter that held back bacteria. Six years later, and without knowledge of the Russian's work, Martines William Beijerinck also found this virus to be filterable, and called it "contagium vivum fluidum" (Hughes, 1977). Much later, but of fundamental importance to the sizing of viruses, was the development of graded membrane filters by Elford in 1931. The earliest classification of viruses was based on sizing by this method. Later, morphological and biochemical methods became available for classification.

Today, these are being replaced by molecular techniques by which the genomic properties and amino acid sequences can be determined.

Electron Microscope

The first electron microscope was built in 1932 by Knoll and Ruska, and the first pictures of a virus, that of tobacco mosaic virus, were shown in 1939 by Kausche *et al.* Over time, and with improvement in techniques, almost all human and animal viruses have been visualized with the electron microscope. The exceptions to this are the slow or unconventional viruses, which are now referred to as "prions" because the infectious particle appears to be a protein rather than a nucleic acid (RNA or DNA), which characterizes conventional viruses. These prion agents cause a number of diseases of animals and man, including a spongioform encephalopathy of sheep (scrapie), mink, and cattle, and kuru, Creutzfeldt–Jakob disease, and Gerstmann–Straussler–Schenker syndrome in humans.

Through the development of methods in preparation, such as metal shadowing, negative staining, freezing, and osmic acid fixation, the morphological appearance of the external surfaces of conventional viruses and bacteria became well characterized under the electron microscope. Plaque counting techniques permitted quantitation of their numbers, and the addition of specific immune sera, which resulted in clumping, allowed specific identification of viral groups (termed "immunoelectron microscopy" or "direct virology" when applied to clinical specimens). Most of these studies involved known viruses that had been identified by other techniques.

The electron microscope has also been the means of discovering new viruses, or at least, of first visualizing viruses suspected of causing a disease, but in which the web of causation was indirect. Two examples of the former will be given and one of the latter.

In 1964, Epstein, Achong, and Barr reported the presence of viral particles under the electron microscope in cultures of lymphoblasts derived from Burkitt's lymphoma, a childhood tumor of African children first described in detail by Denis Burkitt, an English surgeon. The particles were found to be a new herpesvirus, distinct from herpes simplex, varicella/zoster, and cytomegalovirus. It was eventually called Epstein–Barr virus (EBV). While identified in Burkitt tumor tissue, its causal relationship to this tumor remained unclear until added means of identifying the presence of EBV or its antibody became available. The latter technique was provided by Gertrude and Werner Henle in 1966 when they developed an immunofluorescence test for identifying IgG antibody to the viral capsid antigen. This led to both case–control and prospective studies that implicated EBV as an initiator of the pathogenesis of the tumor by creating a proliferation of B lymphocytes. This was augmented by malaria, which is also a B-cell mitogen and also impairs the immune system in its responses to such proliferation. The rapid multiplication of B cells resulted in a chromosomal translocation (from chromosome 8 to chromosome 14, 2, or 22), and with this the activation of an oncogene, c-*myc*, which was the final step in the appearance of a malignant cell whose multiplication constituted Burkitt's lymphoma (Evans and de The, 1989).

The discovery of the immunofluoresence test for EBV also led in 1968 to the discovery by the Henles and Volker Diehl (1968) that EBV was the cause of infectious mononucleosis. It is ironic that Werner Henle was the grandson of Jacob Henle, who proposed the first criteria for causation of an infectious disease in 1840 (see Henle, 1938), yet none of these criteria were met by his grandson in establishing the proof that EBV caused infectious mononucleosis. Indeed, neither EBV nor hepatitis B virus fulfilled the preexisting postulates of Henle–Koch (Henle, 1938; Koch, 1882a; 1936), Rivers (1937), or Huebner (1957). They required new ones based on immunological evidence (Evans, 1974) consisting of (1) the appearance of specific antibody to the agent during the course of the disease, (2) that such immunity protected against primary infection, (3) that only persons lacking the antibody were susceptible to the infection, and (4) that no other antibody could induce similar immunological events.

Another important group of viruses discovered by means of the electron microscope were the rotaviruses. These were identified in duodenal cells and stools of children with acute gastroenteritis in Australia by Bishop and associates (Bishop *et al.*, 1973, 1974). Proof of causation rested on regular identification of the virus in sick children and the appearance of virus-specific antibody. Experimental reproduction of the clinical disease in animals was not possible, and even initial isolation in tissue cultures was extremely difficult. The demonstration by immunoelectron microscopy of both virus and antibody was necessary for viral identification until easier methods, such as radioimmunoassay and ELISA (enzyme-linked immunosorbent assay), were developed. It is now recognized that this group of rotaviruses is the cause of 30–50% of worldwide cases of acute gastroenteritis in children under 3 years old. Vigorous attempts to develop a vaccine with attenuated human strains or animal rotaviruses (the so-called Jennerian approach) are under way. Unfortunately, the diversity of rotavirus strains and their poor antigenic properties are making this a difficult task. Enough evidence of homotypic protection from a vaccine is at hand, however, to indicate fulfillment of Huebner's criterion for causation, i.e., that a vaccine prepared from the putative cause should decrease the incidence of the disease (Huebner, 1957).

For hepatitis A, the electron microscope was the means of establishing visually the presence of a virus in stool samples by Feinstone *et al.* (1973), as well as providing a means of diagnosis by immune electron microscopy. This confirmed epidemiological evidence derived from human volunteer experiments that the virus was present in the stool of infected persons. Attempts to reproduce the disease in nonhuman primates had failed (although infection occurred), as had many early attempts to grow the virus in tissue culture. Later, and with much difficulty, it was successfully adapted to growth in tissue culture by Provost and Hilleman (1979). This has paved the way for development of a vaccine, a task now being vigorously pursued with both killed and attenuated viral preparations. At present the outlook looks very good for an effective vaccine that would protect against infection with HAV. Evidence that such a vaccine decreases or eliminates the disease would also provide a final step in the causal proof that HAV causes infectious hepatitis.

Embryonated Eggs and Tissue Cultures

Tissue cultures of rabbit and guinea pig cornea had been shown by Steinhardt *et al.* (1913) to sustain the growth of vaccinia virus, and in the same year, poliomyelitis virus was reported to grow in cultures of spinal ganglia by Levaditi (1913). Neither of these methods was widely adapted, however, because of the difficulty of maintaining the cultures free of bacterial contamination. Control of this problem awaited the discovery of antibiotics. In the meantime, the chicken embryo was discovered to be an important way to cultivate viruses. For example, Woodruff and Goodpasture (1931) showed that fowlpox virus replicated on the chorioallantoic membrane of developing chick embryos. Subsequently, other poxviruses and herpes simplex viruses were cultivated in a similar way, each producing characteristic plaques on the membrane. Many other viruses, such as the myxoviruses (influenza, Newcastle disease virus, and mumps), were also found to grow in the amniotic sac or allantoic cavity of the chick embryo, and many rickettsiae multiplied in the yolk sac. For these microbial agents, the chick embryo was not the initial means of discovery, but was an important medium for diagnosis and for their growth for vaccines.

In 1945, a major breakthrough came in the use of tissue cultures when Enders *et al.* (1945) reported the growth of poliovirus in tissue cultures derived from various human embryonic sources, for which work they were awarded the Nobel Prize in 1954. Primary kidney cultures were also shown capable of supporting the growth of poliovirus and were the main source of cells for polio vaccines. The addition of antibiotics to their cultures had prevented bacterial and fungal contamination. The use of tissue cultures rapidly expanded from this point onwards. However, these two early tissue culture cells did not grow continuously, and thus required fresh material for every new viral passage. Other cell lines derived from human (HeLa, Hep-2, WI-38) and animal sources (Vero) were then developed and shown to multiply continuously in culture. They provided appropriate substrates for growth of many viruses and for the production of many vaccines. The WI-38 cell line, in particular, was used for many vaccines because it was derived from normal human embryonic lung tissue and did not pose the potential oncogenic problem of introducing cell lines derived from a human malignancy or from an animal source into humans.

Tissue cultures of various sorts also led to the discovery of many new viruses. These included several viruses that cause acute respiratory infections, such as rhinoviruses, adenoviruses, parainfluenza viruses, and respiratory syncytial virus, and also of viruses causing acute infections of the central nervous system, such as the large group of enteroviruses, and of some Coxsackie viruses. The tissue culture systems also provided a method of isolating and propagating exanthem viruses, such as measles and rubella for vaccine production. Vero cells from green monkey kidneys were also an important growth medium for arboviruses.

The evidence for causal associations of these new viruses with the clinical conditions from which they had been isolated came primarily from such viral isolation, as well as the specific antibody responses to them. Reproduction of these diseases in laboratory animals proved very difficult, except for polioviruses, arboviruses, and measles virus [which had been shown capable of producing a rash in monkeys as early as 1921 (Blake and Trask, 1921)].

In 1967 I published a list of "Five Realities of Acute Respiratory Disease" (see Table 3.3) (Evans, 1967) to indicate that (1) the same syndrome could be produced by several agents, (2) the same virus could produce several clinical syndromes, (3) the cause of the syndrome varied by geographic area, age, and other factors, (4) the causes of only about one-half of the common acute respiratory and intestinal syndromes and of about one quarter of acute viral infections of the central nervous system have been identified, and (5) diagnosis of the etiological agent could rarely be made on clinical grounds alone and required laboratory methods such as isolation of the virus and/or demonstration of an antibody response. These same concepts were found later to apply to many syndromes of infectious and chronic diseases as well as to many malignancies. These observations meant that a given virus or bacterium might be established as the cause of a given disease in one setting, but that in another geographic area or another age group, some other infectious agent might result in the same clinical picture.

More recently, the growth of human B and T lymphocytes in suspension cultures has led to the discovery of several important groups of viruses. B-type lymphocytes, derived from lymph node biopsies of cases of Burkitt's lymphoma, were successfully grown *in vitro* in both by Epstein and Barr (1964) and by Pulvertaft (1964). As discussed above, examination of such cultured cells under the electron microscope led to the discovery of Epstein–Barr virus (EBV) (Epstein *et al.*, 1964). Indeed, EBV was found to be necessary for the continual growth of B lymphocytes in the laboratory, their so-called "immortalization."

This virus infects B cells at a receptor site on the cell similar to the receptor of C3 complement.

T-type lymphocytes were more difficult to culture, but were found to multiply in the presence of T-cell growth factor. This led to the discovery of five human retroviruses, originally designated as human T-cell lymphotropic viruses. The first of these, HTLV-I, was isolated by Poiesz *et al.* (1980) and is the cause of adult T-cell leukemia, as well as of tropical spastic paraparesis (Gessain *et al.*, 1985). It occurs primarily in Japan and in the Caribbean islands.

HTLV-II was isolated in 1982 from T cells of a patient with a T-cell variant of hairy cell leukemia (Kalyanaraman *et al.*, 1982). Its full clinical spectrum is unknown.

HTLV-III (now called human immunodeficiency virus or HIV-1) was isolated from lymphocytes of patients with AIDS by Montagnier and his group in France in 1983 (Barre-Sinoussi *et al.*, 1983) and in 1984 by Gallo and associates at the National Institutes of Health in the United States (Gallo *et al.*, 1984). The virus has been propagated in large amounts in special lymphocyte cultures, also developed in Gallo's laboratory in 1984 (Popovic *et al.*, 1984). This has permitted extensive work on the biological, biochemical, and genetic makeup of the virus.

While HIV is widely regarded as the cause of AIDS, and this belief is the basis of our national prevention campaign, a vigorous and outspoken opponent of this view is Peter Duesberg, a distinguished molecular virologist at the University of California, Berkeley (Duesberg, 1987, 1989a). Duesberg's major objections, included in his first paper in 1987, are listed in Table 7.3, to which I have replied in detail (Evans, 1989a). Duesberg then responded to my article in a letter to the journal (Duesberg, 1989b), stating that we agreed on six areas, but disagreed on two, to which I answered that we still disagreed on the concept that HIV led to AIDS and that interruption of virus transmission should decrease the

Table 7.3
Duesberg's Objections to the Concept That HIV Causes Aids[a]

1. Infections with no or low risk for AIDS indicate the virus is not sufficient to cause AIDS.
2. The long incubation period of AIDS is incompatible with the short latent period of viral replication.
3. Levels of AIDS virus expression and infiltration appear too low to account for AIDS or other diseases.
4. AIDS virus is not directly cytocidal.
5. AIDS virus is an indicator of a low risk for AIDS.

[a]Derived from Duesberg (1987).

incidence of the disease (Evans, 1989b). Other scientists have also presented evidence against Duesberg's hypothesis (Blattner *et al.*, 1989; Ginsberg, 1988), but he remains firm in his belief that HIV is not the cause of AIDS (in fact, has nothing to do with it, even as a cofactor) and continues to add detailed virological and epidemiological "evidence" in support of his view (Duesberg, 1990, 1991).

HTLV-IV, now designated as HIV-2, has also been isolated in lymphocyte culture by Clavel *et al.* (1986; see Blattner, 1989) and by Kanki *et al.* (1986), and is another cause of AIDS, although not as pathogenic to the immune system as HIV (Blattner, 1989).

In addition to the retroviruses, a new herpesvirus, originally called human B-lymphotropic virus (HBLV), and now termed human herpes virus type 6 (HHV-6), has been isolated, initially from lymphocytes of a case of AIDS, and subsequently from healthy donors, infants with exanthem subitum, and patients with the chronic fatigue syndrome (Salahuddin *et al.*, 1986, 1988). It can multiply in both B and T lymphocytes. The prevalence of antibody to this virus has been on the order of 60% in healthy donors, indicating it is a very common and often asymptomatic infection. A true causal relationship to primary infection with the virus appears to exist for exanthem subitum (roseola infantum), a common, febrile rash in young children, and with rare cases of an infectious mononucleosis-like syndrome in young adults (Salahuddin *et al.*, 1986). The virus is easily reactivated and antibody has been found in high titer in 80% or so of a number of chronic and malignant conditions, such as chronic fatigue syndrome, Hodgkin's disease, African Burkitt's lymphoma, and acute lymphocytic leukemia. In most of these disease settings, the presence of high antibody titers appears to represent asymptomatic reactivation of the virus and not a primary causal association.

Laboratory Animals

Animal species of all types and sizes have been used for the induction of infection and disease by bacteria and viruses ever since the early work of Klebs and Koch with tuberculosis and anthrax, and of Pasteur with rabies. In his 1955 book on animal viruses, Burnet presents a table listing the animal species employed in the study of 19 viruses, beginning with the 1879 inoculation of rabbits with rabies virus by Galtier, and ending with the isolation of Coxsackie viruses in 1948 by Dalldorf and Sickles (Burnet, 1955). The latter is of particular importance because this was the means by which this group of viruses was first found, and raised the problem of causal association with patients with a nonparalytic polio-like disease, from which it was first isolated. Members of the Coxsackie group have now been shown to be the cause of a wide variety of clinical syndromes involving the central nervous system, respiratory tract, skin, and diaphragmatic pleura (Burnet, 1955).

Another example of the first identification of an agent in an experimental animal is that of kuru, a chronic and fatal degenerative disease of the central nervous system occurring in natives of the Fore tribe in New Guinea. In 1966 Gajdusek and his group at the National Institutes of Health successfully transmitted the disease to chimpanzees (Gajdusek *et al.*, 1966). The transmission of this disease in humans was associated with cannibalism (see Chapter 4). By inoculation of brain material from cases of this disease into chimpanzees, they were able to reproduce the disease clinically and pathologically after a long incubation period. The pathological picture resembled a sponge, so that the name spongioform encephalopathies has been applied to this group of agents. The long incubation period led to the term "slow viruses," and the lack of DNA or RNA in the agents, their high resistance to heat and chemicals, and their failure to induce a demonstrable antibody response resulted in the designation "unconventional viruses." The infectious particle appears to be a form of protein called "prion," and the term "prion" diseases has been suggested for this group, rather than "viruses" because they lack the nucleic acids characteristic of all conventional viruses. The cause of a similar condition, Creutzfeldt–Jakob disease, also produced a similar clinical and pathological disease in chimpanzees and other experimental animals. The finding that these infectious agents could produce chronic degenerative infections of the central nervous system of humans was a key discovery, significant enough for Gajdusek to receive the Nobel Prize. Because these agents could not be grown in tissue culture, nor antibody to them demonstrated, they gave rise to a new set of guidelines for causation. These were published by Johnson and Gibbs (1974) (see Table 4.2). The guidelines were based on the reproducibility and serial transmission of the disease in an experimental animal in several laboratories, and the exclusion of other possible agents contaminating the material.

Other Laboratory Techniques

The agar gel immunodiffusion method for demonstrating precipitin bands that form when antigen and antibody interact was the key technique that permitted Blumberg *et al.* (1965) to discover a new antigen found in the blood of Australian aborigines. Initially, it was called "Australia antigen" because it was not known what disease, if any, was associated with its presence. Subsequent epidemiological and clinical studies by Prince (Prince, 1968) established the virus, hepatitis B virus (HBV), as the cause of a type of hepatitis formerly called "serum" or "transfusion-associated" hepatitis, but now known to be transmitted by parenteral routes, by close contact, and from infected mothers to their offspring. When infection with this virus occurs early in life, as is true in Africa and Asia, the antigen persists in the blood and leads to cirrhosis of the liver and to hepatocellular carcinoma. For his discovery, Blumberg was awarded the Nobel Prize in 1976.

New molecular techniques involving DNA probes, and more recently, the polymerase chain reaction (PCR), are revolutionizing our basic tools in micro-biology (Eisenstein, 1990). They provide very powerful and highly sensitive techniques for identifying antigen in human tissues. Use of PCR, for example, has identified EBV in tissues from Hodgkin's disease (Herbst *et al.,* 1990). The method is being employed to identify the presence of small amounts of viral, bacterial, and parasitic antigens in various tissues, including blood (Eisenstein, 1990). For example, it has permitted the identification of HIV in the blood of 90% of AIDS patients, even well before antibody appears. It is also present in some infants born of HIV-infected mothers, and provides a method to indicate that the infant is infected, since it is impossible to determine for 6 months or so if the antibody in the infant was derived from the mother, or the result of active infection of the newborn. However, the method is currently too complex and expensive for such routine diagnostic tests. The PCR technique is based on amplification of impure DNA by simple chemical proliferation *in vitro* of a predetermined stretch of DNA (Eisenstein, 1990). The method is capable of amplifying specific DNA sequences to more than a millionfold in only a few hours by an automated procedure. At a practical level, it is being applied to the diagnosis of both viral and bacterial infections, as well as to the search for known viral antigens in cancer tissues, such as HTLV-I in T-cell lymphomas, EBV in various lymphomas, hepatitis B and C viruses in liver cancer, and papillomavi-ruses in cervical cancer (Evans and Mueller, 1990). The high sensitivity of the technique also leads to some false-positive reactions, especially cross contamina-tion from true positive samples that have been previously tested in the same laboratory. Careful washing of equipment is essential. While an extremely im-portant method of seeking known microorganisms, the requirement of prior knowledge of a DNA fragment of the infectious agent under study for amplifica-tion limits its application to known agents with known DNA sequences.

Immunology

A key element in establishing that an infectious agent causes a particular disease is the demonstration of the appearance of a specific antibody to the agent, or of a fourfold increase in antibody titer, if antibody is already present when the specimen is taken. The presence of agent-specific IgM antibody is usually indic-ative of a primary infection, although certain reactivated infections, such as cytomegalovirus, are accompanied by a small IgM response. Another highly important discovery is the development of techniques for producing quantities of highly specific monoclonal antibodies, which was first published by Kohler and Milstein (1975). The application of monoclonal antibodies to viral diagnosis has greatly enhanced demonstration of the specificity of the immune response, permitting differentiation between strains of the same agent and of differentiation of a reactivated infection from one due to exogenous reinfection.

Another important arm of the immune response is that of cell-mediated or T-cell immunity, which is demonstrable by skin tests, and is useful in the clinical diagnosis of infection due to agents that cannot be grown in culture and/or for which a demonstrable antibody response is not produced. The organism that causes leprosy, *M. leprae,* is an example.

This section will briefly review the history of the key developments and is derived from Bulloch (1938), Foster (1970), and Bellanti (1988). Only key original references derived from these sources will be cited.

Antibodies and the Immune Response

The observation by Edward Jenner that persons who got well after cowpox were immune to smallpox led to his introduction of cowpox vaccine in 1798 (Jenner, 1798). This was an empiric discovery without scientific basis at the time, but the concept on which it was based has withstood the test of time and has eventually led to the complete eradication of smallpox from the world in 1977. About 100 years after Jenner's publication, Louis Pasteur and his associates began the scientific approach to immunology by preparing attenuated strains of microorganisms for protection against infectious diseases, first with fowl cholera vaccine in 1878–1880 (Pasteur, 1880) and then with anthrax in 1881 (Pasteur *et al.,* 1881). Based on Jenner's contribution, Pasteur coined the term "vaccine" (from *vacca,* Latin for cow) for these immunizations. The use of these living attenuated, as well as heat-killed cultures for prophylaxis against infectious diseases constitutes *active* immunization. The proof that this type of immunity, called *humoral* immunity, was due to antibody production was the sentinel observation of Behring and Kitasato (1890). They demonstrated the neutralizing antitoxic activity of sera from animals immunized with tetanus toxin, who were protected against infection. This was followed one week later by a paper by Behring showing the same to be true of diphtheria toxin. In their joint paper, it was also shown that the neutralizing activity of tetanus antitoxin could be transferred by serum from immunized animals to uninoculated animals and to result in protection, a process now known as *passive* immunization. In 1895, Calmette published evidence of the neutralizing property in snake venom antiserum (Calmette, 1895). A mechanism to explain how antibody is produced and how it acts was proposed by Paul Ehrlich in 1897, and was termed the "side chain" or "receptor" theory (Ehrlich, 1897).

After viruses were discovered, it was found that the production of a demonstrable, specific immune antibody response occurred much more frequently in viral than in bacterial diseases, and constituted a critical element of viral diagnosis. An important test to demonstrate humoral antibodies was the complement fixation test developed by Bordet and Gengou (1901), but it was much later when Rivers (1937) suggested that the appearance of specific antibody during a viral infection constituted an important element in establishing causation. This was reaffirmed in the guidelines suggested by Huebner (1957) for proof of causation in a viral disease. He also added the concept that longitudinal epidemiological studies were helpful in establishing causation, as was the demonstration that protection against infection followed the use of a vaccine prepared using the candidate causal agent. Later, for infections like EBV in infectious mononucleosis and HBV in viral hepatitis, in which the causative agent could not be grown in the laboratory, the demonstration of an immune response to the candidate agent constituted the major basis for causal inferences. These criteria were published by Evans (1974).

In addition to humoral immunity, an important arm of protection against infection is that termed *cell-mediated immunity,* or in more modern terminology, B- and T-cell immunity. On a practical basis, the most common method to demonstrate the presence of this type of immunity is a skin test, in which a small amount of the antigen is inoculated intracutaneously and followed for 24–72 hours for the appearance of an indurated, red reaction at the site of injection. Perhaps the first demonstration of this phenomenon and of its use as a diagnostic test was the tuberculin test for tuberculosis (Koch, 1890). Cell-mediated immunity (CMI) is important in the control of viruses, fungi, bacteria, and other intracellular parasites. CMI is demonstrable through the skin test, and this is used in the diagnosis of infections, such as tuberculosis and leprosy, in which no antibody response is demonstrable. However, to my knowledge it has not been included as a criterion of causal proof of an infectious disease. For this reason, further historical discussion of its development will not be pursued.

References

Barre-Sinoussi F, Chermann JC, Rey F, *et al:* Isolation of a T-lymphotropic deficiency syndrome (AIDS). *Science* **220:**868–871, 1983.

Behring E von, Kitasato S: Ueber das Zustandekommen des Diphtherie-Immunitat und des Tetanus-Immunitat bei Thieren. *Dtsch Med Wochenschr* **16:**1113–1114, 1890.

Bellanti JA: *Immunology III.* W B Saunders, Philadelphia, 1988.

Bishop RF, Davidson GP, Holmes IH, *et al:* Viral particle in epithelial cells of duodenal mucosa from children with acute gastroenteritis. *Lancet* **2:**128–183, 1973.

Bishop RF, Holmes IH, Ruck BJ: Detection of a new virus by electron microscopy of fecal extracts of children with gastroenteritis. *Lancet* **1:**149–151, 1974.

Blake FC, Trask JD: Studies on measles. II. Symptomatology and pathology in monkeys experimentally infected. *J Exp Med* **33:**413–422, 1921.

Blattner WA: Retroviruses, in Evans AS (ed): *Viral Infection of Humans: Epidemiology and Control.* 3rd ed. New York, Plenum Press, 1989, pp 545–592.

Blattner W, Gallo RC, Temin HM: Blattner and colleagues respond to Duesberg. *Science* **241**:514–515, 1989.

Blumberg BS, Alter HJ, Visnick S: A 'new' antigen in leukemia sera. *JAMA* **191**:541–546, 1965.

Bordet J, Gengou O: Sur l'existence de substance sensibilisatrices dans la plupart des serums anti-microbiens. *Ann Inst Pasteur* **5**:289–303, 1901.

Bulloch W: *The History of Bacteriology.* London, Oxford University Press, 1938.

Burkitt DP: A sarcoma involving the jaws of African children. *Brit J Surg* **46**:218–223, 1958.

Burnet FM: *Principles of Animal Virology.* New York, Academic Press, 1955.

Calmette A: Contributions a l'etude des venims, des toxines et des serum antitoxique. *Ann Inst Pasteur* **9**:225–231, 1895.

Clavel F, Guetard D, Bran-Vezinet FB, *et al:* Isolation of a new human retrovirus from West African patients with AIDS. *Science* **233**:343–346, 1986.

Darling ST: A protozoan general infection producing pseudotuberculosis in the lungs and necrosis of the liver, spleen, and lymph nodes. *JAMA* **466**:1283, 1906.

Dobell C: *Antony van Leeuwenhoek and His Little Animals.* New York, Dover, 1932.

Duesberg P: Retroviruses as carcinogens and pathogens. Expectations and reality. *Cancer Res* **47**:1199–1226, 1987.

Duesberg PH: Human immunodeficiency virus and acquired immunodeficiency syndrome: Correlation but not causation. *Proc Natl Acad Sci USA* **86**:755-764, 1989a.

Duesburg P: Does HIV cause AIDS? *J AIDS* **2**:514–515, 1989b.

Duesberg P: Quantitation of human immunodeficiency virus in the blood (letter). *N Engl J Med* **322**:1466, 1990.

Duesburg PH: AIDS epidemiology: Inconsistencies with human immunodeficiency virus and with infectious disease. *Proc Natl Acad Sci USA* **88**:1575–1579, 1991.

Ehrlich P: Zur Kenntniss des Antitoxinwirking. *Fortschr Med* **15**:41–43, 1897.

Eisenstein BI: Current concepts: The polymerase chain reaction—new method of using medical genetics for medical diagnosis. *N Engl J Med* **322**:178–182, 1990.

Elford WJ: A series of graded membranes suitable for general bacteriological use, especially in filterable virus studies. *J Pathol Bacteriol* **34**:505–552, 1931.

Enders JH, Weller TH, Robbins FC: Cultivation of the Lansing strain of poliomyelitis virus in various human embryonic tissues. *Science* **109**:85–87, 1945.

Epstein MA, Barr YM: Cultivation *in vitro* of human lymphoblasts from Burkitt's lymphoma. *Lancet* **1**:252–253, 1964.

Epstein MA, Achong BG, Barr YM: Virus particles in cultured lymphoblasts from Burkitt's lymphoma. *Lancet* **1**:702–703, 1964.

Evans AS: Clinical syndromes in adults caused by respiratory infection. *Med Clin North Am* **51**:803–815, 1967.

Evans AS: New discoveries in infectious mononucleosis. *Mod Med* **42**:18–24, 1974.

Evans AS: Causation and disease: The Henle–Koch postulates revisited. *Yale J Biol Med* **49**:175–195, 1976.

Evans AS: Limitations to Koch's postulates. *Lancet* **2**:1277–1278, 1977.

Evans AS: Discussion, in Lilienfeld AM (ed): *Time, Places, and Persons: Aspects of the History of Epidemiology.* Baltimore, Johns Hopkins University Press, 1980, pp 94–98.

Evans AS: The clinical illness promotion factor. A third ingredient. *Yale J Biol Med* **55**:193–199, 1985.

Evans AS: Does HIV cause AIDS? An historical perspective. *J AIDS* **2**:107–113, 1989a.

Evans AS: Does HIV cause AIDS: Author's reply (letters to the editor). *J AIDS* **2**:515–517, 1989b.

Evans AS: Epidemiological concepts, in Evans AS, Brachman PS (eds): *Bacterial Infections of Humans: Epidemiology and Control,* 2nd ed. New York, Plenum Press, 1991a, pp 1–57.

Evans AS, de The G: Epstein Barr virus, in Evans AS (ed): *Viral Infections of Humans: Epidemiology and Control,* 3rd ed. New York, Plenum Press, 1989, pp 713–735.

Evans AS, Mueller NE: Viruses and cancer. Causal associations. *Ann Epidemiol* **1:**71–92, 1990.

Evans AS: Causation and disease: Effect of technology on postulates of causation. *Yale J Biol Med* **64:**513–528, 1991b.

Evans AS: Evans' postulates, in: Last JM (ed), *A Dictionary of Epidemiology* (2nd ed). New York, Oxford University Press, 1983, p 44.

Feinstone SM, Kapikian AZ, Purcell RH: Hepatitis A: Detection by immune electron microscopy of a virus-like antigen associated with acute illness. *Science* **182:**1026–1028, 1973.

Fenner F, Gibbs A (eds): *Portraits of Viruses.* Basel, Karger, 1988.

Fenner F, Henderson DA, Arita A, *et al* (eds): *Smallpox and its Eradication.* Geneva, World Health Organization, 1989.

Foster WD: *A History of Bacteriology and Immunology.* Wm Heinemann Medical Books Ltd. London, 1970.

Gajdusek DC, Gibbs CJ Jr, Alpers M: Experimental transmission of a kuru-like syndrome to chimpanzees. *Nature* **209:**794–796, 1966.

Gallo RC, Salahuddin SZ, Popovic M, *et al:* Frequent detection and isolation of cytopathic retroviruses (HTLV-III) from patients with AIDS and at risk for AIDS. *Science* **224:**500–503, 1984.

Gangarosa EJ, Beisel WR, Benyajati C, *et al:* The nature of the gastrointestinal lesion in Asiatic cholera and its relation to pathogenesis. *Am J Trop Med Hyg* **9:**125–135, 1960.

Gessain A, Barin F, Vermont JC, *et al:* Antibodies to human T-lymphotropic virus type-1 in patients with tropical spastic paraparesis. *Lancet* **2:**407–410, 1985.

Ginsberg HA: Scientific forum on AIDS: A summary. Does HIV cause AIDS? *J AIDS* **1:**165–172, 1988.

Hansen GH: On the etiology of leprosy. English translation. Br. and Foreign. *Med Chir* **55:**459, 1875.

Henle G, Henle W: Immunofluorescence in cells derived from Burkitt's lymphoma. *J Bacteriol* **91:**1248–1256, 1966.

Henle G, Henle W, Diehl V: Relation of Burkitt's tumor associated herpes-type virus to infectious mononucleosis. *Proc Natl Acad Sci USA* **59:**94–101, 1968.

Henle J: *On Miasmata and Contagie,* Rosen G (trans). Baltimore, Johns Hopkins University Press, 1938.

Herbst H, Niedobitek G, Kneba M, *et al:* High incidence of Epstein–Barr virus genome in Hodgkin's disease. *Am J Pathol* **137:**13–18, 1990.

Huebner RJ: The virologist's dilemma. *Ann NY Acad Sci* **67:**430–442, 1957.

Hughes SS: *The Virus: A History of the Concept.* London, Heinemann Educational Books, 1977.

Jenner E: An Inquiry into the Causes and Effects of Variolae Vaccine, a Disease Discovered in Some of the Western Counties of England, Particularly Gloustershire and Known by the Name of Cowpox. London, Sampson Low, 1798.

Johnson RT, Gibbs CJ Jr: Editorial. Koch's postulates and slow infections of the nervous system. *Arch Neurol* **30:**36–38, 1974.

Kalyanaraman VS, Sarngadharan MG, Robert-Guroff M, *et al:* Leukemia virus (HTLV-II) associated with a T-cell variant of hairy cell leukemia. *Science* **218:**571, 1982.

Kanki PJ, Barin F, M'Boup S, *et al:* New human T-lymphotropic virus type III (StLV-III AGM) *Science* **232:**238–243, 1986.

Kausche SSA, Pfankuch T, Ruska H: Die Sichtbarmachung von pflanzlichen Virus in Ubermikroscop. *Naturwissenschaften* **27:**292–299, 1939.

Knoll M, Ruska E: Das Electronenmikroskop. *Z Physiol* **78:**31, 1932.

Koch R: Die Atiologie de Tuberkulose. *Berl Klin Wochenschr* **19:**221–230, 1882a.

Koch R: *Uber Die Atiologie Der Tuberkulose.* Verhandlugen des Kongresses fur Inner Medicine. Erste Kongress, Weisbaden, 1882b, Verlag von JF Bergmann, pp 56–66.

Koch R: Uber die Cholerabakterien. *Deutsche Med Wochenschr Berlin* **10:**725–728, 1884.

Koch R: Uber bacteriologische forschung. *Dtsch Med Wochenschr* **16:**756–757, 1890.

Koch R: Uber den augenblicklichen Stand der Bacteriologischen Cholera Diagnose. *J Hyg Infektionskr* **14:**319, 1893.

Koch R: *Die Bekampfung des Typhus. Veroffentlichungen auf dem Gebiete des Militacischen Sanitas-Wessen, Vol. 21.* Berlin, Hirchwald, Gessammelte Werke 2/1, 1903, pp 296–305.

Koch R: *Die aetiologie der milzbrand krankheiten begrunded auf die entwicklungegeschichte des Bacillus anthrasis 1876.* Eingeleitet de M Fischer, Hierzn 1 tafel, JA Barth, 1910.

Koch R: *The Etiology of Anthrax, 1877. The Etiology of Tuberculosis, 1882.* Baltimore, Williams and Wilkins, 1938.

Kohler G, Milstein C: Continuous cultures of fused cells secreting antibody of defined specificity. *Nature* **256:**495–497, 1975.

Ledingham JCG, Arkwright JA: *The Carrier Problem in Infectious Diseases.* London, Longmans Grove 1912.

Levaditi C: Virus de la poliomyelete et culture des cellules *in vitro C R Seances Soc Biol* **75:**202–205, 1913.

Löffler F: Untersuchen uber die Bedeutung der Mikrorganismen fur die Entstehung der Diphtherie beim Menschen, bei Taube und beim Kalbe. *Mitt K GesundhAmt* **2:**421, 1884.

Melany HE: Pulmonary histoplasmosis. Report of two cases. *Am Rev Tuberc* **44:**240–247, 1941.

Mims CA: *The Pathogenesis of Infectious Disease.* New York, Academic Press, 1982.

Park W, Beebe AC: Diphtheria and pseudodiphtheria. *Med Rec* **46:**385–401, 1894.

Pasteur L: Sur les maladies virulentes, et en particulier sur la maladie appelee vulgairement cholera des poules. *C R Acad Sci Ser D* **90:**239, 1880.

Pasteur L, Chamberland C, Roux E: De la possibilite de Rendre Les Moutons Refractaires su Charbon par la methode des inoculations preventives. *C R Acad Sci Ser D* **92:**662–666, 1881.

Poiesz BJ, Ruscetti FW, Gazdar AF, *et al:* Detection and isolation of type-C retrovirus particles from fresh and cultured lymphocytes of patients with cutaneous T-cell lymphomas. *Proc Natl Acad Sci USA* **77:**7415–7419, 1980.

Popovic M, Sarngadharan MG, Read E, *et al:* Detection, isolation, and continuous production of cytopathic retroviruses (HTLV-III) from patients with AIDS and pre-AIDS. *Science* **224:**497–500, 1984.

Prince AM: An antigen detected in the blood during the incubation period of serum hepatitis. *Proc Natl Acad Sci USA* **60:**814–821, 1968.

Provost PJ, Hilleman MR: Propagation of human A hepatitis virus in cell culture *in vitro. Proc Exp Biol Med* **80:**213–221, 1979.

Pulvertaft RJV: Cytology of Burkitt's tumor (African lymphoma). *Lancet* **1:**238–240, 1964.

Reed W, Vaughan VC, Shakespeare EO: *Origin and spread of typhoid fever in U.S. military camps during the Spanish War of 1898.* Washington, DC, 1900–1904, abstract of report.

Rivers TM: Viruses and Koch's postulates. *J Bacteriol* **33:**1–12, 1937.

Salahuddin SZ, Ablashi DV, Markham PD, *et al:* Isolation of a new virus, HBLV, in patients with lymphoproliferative disorders. *Science* **234:**596–601, 1986.

Salahuddin SZ, Ablashi DV, Josephs SF, *et al:* Human herpes-6 (human B-lymphotrophic virus), in Ablashi DV, Fagioni A, Krueger RF, *et al* (eds): *Epstein–Barr Virus and Human Disease.* Clifton, NJ, Humana Press, 1988, pp 461–472.

Soper GA: Typhoid carrier. *JAMA* **48:**2019–2022, 1907.

Soper GA: The curious career of Typhoid Mary. *Bull NY Acad Med* **15:**698–712, 1939.

Steinhardt E, Israelie C, Lambert RA: Studies on the cultivation of the virus of vaccinia. *J Infect Dis* **13:**294-300, 1913.

Woodruff AM, Goodpasture EW: The susceptibility of the chorioallantoic membrane of chick embryos to infection with the fowl-pox virus. *Am J Pathol* **209:**22, 1931.

Challenges to the Epidemiology of Infectious Diseases in the Next Decade

A priority list of the major challenges in human infectious disease epidemiology for the next decade is presented in Table 8.1. The discussion in this chapter of the major items on this list is derived from several recent papers and presentations (Evans, 1985b, 1987, 1989d, 1990; Evans and Brachman, 1986; Shope and Evans, 1989).

Retroviruses

In my view, control of the retrovirus infections of humans—HIV-1 and 2 and HTLV-I—is now and will remain our major challenge in the decade or so to come.

In 1988, the infectious diseases occupying the most space in two of the most prominent journals, the *New England Journal of Medicine* and *The Lancet,* were AIDS, leading the list, followed by viral hepatitis, herpes infections, and malaria (Table 8.2). Many papers dealt with the virus itself, the human immunodeficiency virus (HIV-1), which destroys the immune system and leads to the syndrome of AIDS. While doubts on the necessary and sufficient role of this virus in the causation of AIDS have been raised by a prominent virologist, Dr. Peter Duesberg (1987, 1988), there is no question in my mind that public health policy must be based on control of HIV transmission, if we are to reduce the impact of this dreadful epidemic. A related virus, designated as HIV-2, also can lead to AIDS and is the predominant infection in certain parts of Africa. Given the current and projected number of persons with AIDS and HIV infection (Table 8.3), one can predict that these topics will dominate our journals, our medical and hospital

Table 8.1
Priorities for the Epidemiology of Infectious Diseases in the Next Decade

1. Control of retroviruses (HIV-1, HIV-2, HTLV-I)
2. Control of other high-incidence infections
3. Expand and improve immunization programs
4. Recognition and control of new infectious agents
5. Early diagnosis and detection of epidemic diseases
6. Improvement in surveillance in developed and developing countries including surveillance of animal and avian diseases
7. Apply molecular techniques to epidemiology and control of infectious diseases and to their pathogenesis
8. Train more epidemiologists, especially for developing countries, and in epidemiology, molecular biology, and genetics in developed countries for future challenges
9. Expand the concept of the hospital epidemiologist to the outpatient department and the clinics
10. Seek to understand the pathogenesis of disease both in the community and in the individual as a basis for prevention

practice, our health insurance, our national costs for health care, as well as many other aspects of our society over the next decade or longer. For example, over 100,000 cases have been reported in the first 8 years (1981–1989) and a second 100,000 during the next 2 years (September 1989–November 1991) (MMWR, 1989, 1991, 1992). Even if all transmission were to cease today, there are an estimated 1 million persons in the United States already infected with HIV, most of whom will fall ill and die over the next decade. Some 76% of those infected have developed AIDS or related manifestations 7 years after infection. With an average incubation period of 11.5 years, more can be expected to do so later. While there will be a declining incidence in homosexuals, that in I.V. drug users, heterosexual contacts of current cases, and infants of infected mothers will continue to rise and produce wide and profound effects on our health care system and on the very fabric of our society in endemic areas. The worldwide picture is equally alarming with over 375,000 cases reported currently and 10 million infected. By the year 2000, it is estimated that the cumulative number of clinical AIDS cases will total 10 million adults and 5 million children (Mann, 1992). It is imperative that countries where HIV has not spread, or is just emerging, mount extensive educational programs on how the virus is transmitted and on ways to prevent it. Asia is a high priority in this regard in my view. The pernicious circle of drug addiction (especially cocaine and crack), poverty, crime, and prostitution of both males and females must not be allowed to establish itself globally, as it has in urban centers of the United States and many other centers of the developed world, as well as throughout much of Africa. HIV is also invading our college populations and vigorous educational efforts must be carried out now, led by the students themselves. Our national programs must not be directed at HIV alone, but at the wider and more acceptable aim of control of all sexual and blood-borne diseases (Evans, 1988). These now include HIV, HTLV-I, hepatitis A, B, and C, syphilis, Epstein–Barr virus, and cytomegalovirus. There is a growing threat of HTLV-I in I.V. drug users, which can lead to adult T-cell leukemia, tropical spastic paraparesis, and perhaps other diseases. HTLV-I may amplify the growth of HIV, since it infects the same cells. Also benefitting from such widened programs would be not only the prevention of other venereal infections such as genital herpes and syphilis, which become more severe in HIV-infected persons, and both gonorrhea and nongonorrheal urethritis, but also the spread of HIV itself. The penile lesions of herpes and syphilis provide entry for the virus and the discharge of urethritis carries HIV-infected leukocytes with it. Nonvenereal diseases would also benefit by a widened program. The most serious of these is tuberculosis, whose incidence, clinical severity, and drug resistance are rapidly increasing in HIV-infected persons. Skin tests and chest X-rays of all AIDS

Table 8.2
Number of Papers Devoted to Infectious Disease Subjects in the *New England Journal of Medicine* and *The Lancet* in 1988[a]

New England Journal of Medicine (Jan.–Dec., 1988)		*Lancet* (Jan.–July, 1988)	
1. AIDS and ARC	62	1. HIV	76
2. HIV	54	2. AIDS	44
3. Herpesviruses	8	3. Herpesviruses	29
EBV	4	EBV	1
CMV	3	CMV	17
HSV	1	HSV	9
		HHV-6	12
4. Japanese B encephalitis and vaccine	5	4. Hepatitis	23
5. HTLV-I	4	5. Malaria	14
6. Malaria	4	6. Legionnaire's	10
7. Tuberculosis	4	7. Salmonella	7
8. Hepatitis	4	8. HTLV-I	5
9. Meningococcal dis.	3	9. Listerosis	5
10. Legionella	3	10. Measles	3

[a]From Evans (1990).

Table 8.3
HIV Infections and AIDS as of December 1991

United States (CDC, 1992)
Total cases $(6/1981-12/1991) = 206,392^a$

	First 100,000 (6/1981-8/1989)	Second 100,000 (9/1989-12/1991)
	Percent distribution of cases	
Transmission		
Homosexual/bisexual	61	55
I.V. drug users	20	24
Heterosexual	5	7
Transfusion	2.5	1.9
Gender		
Males	91	88
Females	9	12
Race		
Black	27	31
Hispanic	15	17

HIV infections
Estimated number = 1 million; 20% have developed AIDS. About half of those infected meet current CDC surveillance case definition of AIDS (CD4 counts < 200,000 ML.)

Global (Mann, 1992)
Estimated number infected = 10 million (Africa, 6 million; North and South America, 1 million each; Europe, 1/2 million). Estimated number with AIDS by the year 2000 = 10 million adults, 5 million children.

^{a}Deaths = 133,232.

patients and their contacts will be needed to control this serious threat. Methadone clinics for I.V. drug users should also be prepared to check for both HIV and tuberculosis and to have antituberculosis drugs on hand. Special isolation facilities will be needed and the old isolation sanitaria reactivated. Effective transmission of the other infections that are spread by the same routes, including HBV, is needed since HBV is said to be some ten times more infectious than

HIV. Animal models are desperately needed to judge the effectiveness of new therapies and new approaches to prevention such as CD4 receptor-blocking agents, interferon, and other immunological modalities. Mouse and nonhuman primate models are now appearing. As of this writing, the antigenic diversity of HIV, its ability to coexist in the presence of antibody, and the fact that it attacks the key cells that are responsible for mounting an immune response against an infectious agent, all make the possibility of an effective vaccine rather remote. Indeed, evidence now suggests that variation in the virus during a single human passage may lead to one that escapes our normal immune mechanisms, and which becomes more lytic for CD4 T cells, leading to the development of AIDS. The diversity of these emerging mutants in the same individual is another block to effective vaccine development. Even if a vaccine were available today, it would be difficult to identify and protect all of the persons at highest risk, and to convince them to use the vaccine in view of the difficulty in altering their behavioral patterns that led to infection. This would be especially true of the I.V. drug users. The homosexual groups in large cities seem much better organized and susceptible to changes in their behavioral patterns.

Other Infectious Agents

In addition to the retroviruses, one can predict that attention over the next decade will be given to hepatitis B virus (HBV), its inclusion in routine immunization programs, and its use at birth in developing countries in the hopes of preventing hepatocellular carcinoma. Hepatitis B control would also prevent Delta hepatitis (HDV), since it is dependent on HBV for its carriage and multiplication. Non-A non-B hepatitis, parenteral or type-B-like, which is now designated as hepatitis C virus (HCV), will demand increasing efforts for its screening in blood banks, for its spread by I.V. drug users, and eventually for a vaccine, if it can be grown in tissue culture, or its infectious RNA isolated, inactivated, and inserted into an appropriate carrier particle. This virus is responsible for 80% of transfusion-associated hepatitis in developed countries and can lead to chronic liver disease, cirrhosis, and hepatocellular carcinoma (Evans and Mueller, 1990); tests for antibody detection are now commercially available and a double polymerase chain reaction (PCR) test for antigen detection is under development.

The herpesvirus infections will continue to be a challenge. This includes the newly discovered type 6 (HHV-6), which is now recognized as responsible for exanthem subitum and some cases of mono-like illness. The virus infects almost everyone at a young age and is readily reactivated in conditions of immunodeficiency. EBV, already implicated in the pathogenesis of African Burkitt's lymphoma and nasopharyngeal carcinoma, presents altered, but different, antibody patterns, some years before the development of Hodgkin's disease (Mueller *et al.*, 1989) and of non-Hodgkin's lymphoma (Mueller *et al.*, 1991). Whether these findings represent true causal connections or are simply markers for perturbations in the immune system that lead to the emergence of a malignant cell awaits careful molecular and epidemiological investigation. Papillomavirus will be of increasing concern in relation to cervical cancer, but better molecular differentiation of viral types and the development of a type-specific monoclonal antibody test will be needed to evaluate its causal relation to cancer of the cervix, rectal carcinoma, and other epithelial cancers. Such technical advances are on the horizon, but a vaccine that can be shown to reduce the risk of these malignancies may be needed to establish firm causal evidence (Evans and Mueller, 1990). Leading workers in the field, such as Dr. Harold Zur Hausen, feel even now that papillomaviruses are necessary but insufficient causes of these malignancies (Zur Hausen, 1991). Human T-cell leukemia/lymphoma virus has a very strong causal relationship to adult T-cell leukemia (ATL) and tropical spastic paraparesis, and perhaps to other chronic infections of the central nervous system. It will be of increasing public health concern not only in Japan and the Caribbean where it is already well established, but also in the United States and other countries where the virus is invading the blood supply via I.V. drug users or is passed along to the offspring via breast milk from mothers infected with the virus.

An increasing spectrum of HIV-related malignant and chronic diseases will be seen by oncologists and neurologists. Search for the cause or causes of the chronic fatigue syndrome will probably be with us for some time but it is unlikely that EBV will be among them (Gold *et al.*, 1990; Evans, 1991); stress and depression are closely associated with the syndrome but whether cause or effect will remain an enigma. The elusive cause or causes of Kawasaki disease or syndrome have thus far resisted vigorous microbiological and immunological investigation (Evans, 1989b,c). Early evidence that a new retrovirus or EBV might be causally related has not been confirmed in subsequent studies. Perhaps the polymerase chain reaction for EBV and other agents may yield clues, as will bacterial "superantigens" that evoke vigorous immune responses. This unusual exanthem and mucous membrane disease of Japan, Hawaii, and now of many other countries in lesser incidence, is of great pathogenetic and epidemiological interest because of its essential limitation to very young children, its apparent epidemic occurrence in Japan without evidence of person-to-person spread, and the delayed occurrence of aneurysms of the coronary arteries in 15–20% of the infected children in a manner suggestive of an autoimmune phenomenon.

Among bacterial infections, Lyme disease, now achieving epidemic levels in many states, Legionnaire's disease, *Mycoplasma pneumonia* infections, gonorrhea, chlamydia infections of the eye and genital tract, and pneumonia in infants and young adults (TWAR strain) will all be of increasing concern over the next decade because there is no vaccine for any of these, and because control of the transmission of respiratory and sexually transmitted infections is so difficult. Veterinary research on tick control, the avian spread of *Borrelia burgdorferi,* the causative agent of Lyme disease, and efforts at vaccine development for both humans and domestic animals are challenges in the widening spread of Lyme disease by ticks, and of hysteria by the vector of the news media. Some encouraging results with a vaccine for dogs and cats are now emerging. Perhaps this will lead to a human vaccine for high-risk persons by the end of the next decade. Standardization and improvement in the current diagnostic tests for Lyme disease are badly needed. Tuberculosis remains an unmet challenge, one responsible before AIDS for about 40% of deaths from infectious diseases in the United States. As discussed above, it is now one of the diseases on the rise in conjunction with HIV infections, both in the extent and the severity of clinical illness in persons with either primary or reactivated infections. Where is the next generation of BCG vaccines? Where are drugs that are effective against new drug resistant strains?

Diarrhea will remain a global problem over the next decade, especially in developing countries. Vigorous promotion of UNICEF oral water replacement salts will be necessary along with the new knowledge that several cereal grains can replace glucose in the oral formulations. Trials of several rotavirus vaccines are in progress. To date, however, the antigenic diversity of the rotaviruses has been a major problem in vaccine effectiveness, including strains derived from both animal and human sources.

The incidence of slow viral infections will be increasing through organ transplants and in HIV-infected persons. Creutzfeldt–Jakob disease (CJD) has been transmitted via growth hormone derived from human pituitary glands as well as from dural tissue stored in a tissue bank in Germany. This group of viruses produce spongioform encephalitis, contain no DNA or RNA, fail to mount an immune response, and are extremely resistant to chemicals, heat, and ultraviolet light. They are infectious in very high titers and much is known of their point mutations and amino acid sequences. They may be self-replicating agents (Brown *et al.,* 1991; Gajdusek, 1990). Slow viral infections of animals, such as the wide spread of bovine spongioform encephalopathy in England, are producing severe economic problems there. The worldwide infection of sheep, goats, and mink with scrapie virus is not only an economic problem, but means that these unconventional viruses are entering the human food chain through use of materials from such infected species in animal food supplements and in sausages prepared for human consumption (Gajdusek, 1990). The fact that the incidence of CJD is 1 in a million in each country of the world suggests the possibility of wide exposure to slow viruses but with only a very rare clinically expressed disease, perhaps on a genetic basis. About 5% of cases are clearly familial with a defined pattern of an autosomal dominant disease. Progressive multifocal leukoencephalophy (PLM), due to the JC strain of papovavirus that infects most children early in life and leads to a latent infection without known primary clinical manifestations, is reactivated and producing clinical illness in about 4% of AIDS patients whereas it was a rare disease before.

Certainly, malaria and schistosomiasis will be with us for a long time despite great effort to develop vaccines and effective control programs. The drug resistance of *Plasmodium falciparum* has been a continual challenge to pharmaceutical houses although promising results are now appearing.

Immunization Programs

Hopefully, those childhood infections against which WHO's Expanded Program in Immunization (EPI) is directed, namely, diphtheria, pertussis, tetanus, poliomyelitis, measles, and tuberculosis, will be under much better control by the end of this century. The participation of other organizations such as UNICEF, the Rockefeller Foundation, the Child Survival Program and others, offers hope that realistic goals will be met. The need for serologic monitoring and the criteria for control have been discussed elsewhere (Evans, 1980; 1984a, b, c). The major deterrents to success in developing countries are the general problems of getting the mothers to bring the children back for the three to four shots required, the problems of transport of materials and vaccine in difficult terrain, especially in the rainy season, and the maintenance of the cold chain in tropical climates. Specific problems are the difficulty of getting a good antibody response to measles vaccine in the presence of maternal antibody, poor immune response to oral polio vaccine in certain African and other countries, and the need for a better pertussis vaccine. A priority list for improved or needed vaccines for both developing and developed countries was prepared by the National Institute of Allergy and Infectious Diseases (1985) and is shown in Table 8.4. Great progress has

Table 8.4
Vaccine Priorities[a,b]

United States	Developing Countries
1. Hepatitis B	1. *Streptococcus pneumoniae*
2. Respiratory syncytial virus	2. Plasmodia species
3. *Haemophilus influenzae* type B	3. Rotoviruses—3 types
4. Influenza	4. *Salmonella typhii*
5. Varicella-Zoster	5. Shigella species

[a]From National Institute of Allergy and Infectious Diseases (1985).
[b]If technical developments permit, *Streptococcus* Group B and *Neisseria gonorrhoeae* should be placed on the list.

already been made on an HBV vaccine based on HBV DNA insertion into a yeast carrier, and other cheaper vaccines made from carriers are being widely used in developing countries in babies with high hopes of reducing 80% or more of the hepatocellular carcinoma that is associated with prolonged HBV infection. No vaccine is currently is sight for the 10–15% that may be associated with HCV. Promising results with both killed and attenuated HAV vaccines are being obtained in clinical trials, including U.S. Army trials with a killed HAV–HBV vaccine. A much more potent and standardized inactivated poliomyelitis has been developed and field-tested, and is equal in potency to oral vaccine (OPV). It has been found to be immunogenic in geographic areas where OPV has failed (Stoeckel *et al.,* 1984). Its major limitations are that it does not prevent multiplication and spread of wild poliovirus from the gut, and that its cost is presently high. A combination of oral and killed vaccines in such areas may lead to control of both infection and disease through poliomyelitis vaccine, if the cost of production of killed vaccine will permit its use. The next decade should tell us whether WHO's goal of eradicating poliomyelitis from the world will succeed. Indeed, the Pan American Health Association (PAHO) had an even earlier goal, 1990, for the Americas and great progress toward this end had been made with improved potency and larger-dose oral vaccines, better formulation of the types, and, most important, a massive 2-day annual immunization program. We are nearing elimination of paralytic poliomyelitis in the Americas. It should be noted that the oral polio vaccines employed in the EPI programs were of a lesser potency and in a 0.1-ml dose rather than 1.0 ml used in the United States. The difficult logistics of vaccine delivery in Africa, the problems of the rainy season and of maintenance of the cold chain, and the dispersion of the population will be major obstacles toward the true global eradication of poliomyelitis in these settings. True eradication means the elimination of the clinical disease, of the infection, and of the organism in the environment on a global basis (Evans, 1984a,b). I remain skeptical that full eradication of both infection and disease can be accomplished, although I am confident that the prevention of most cases of paralytic poliomyelitis can be achieved (Evans, 1984a,b).

For measles, the major problems in *developing* countries are the maintenance of the cold chain and the need for effective vaccination in settings in which measles often occurs earlier than 9 months of age (the current age of EPI vaccination), or even 6 months of age, at a time when maternal antibody is still present. In response to these problems in developing countries, a more potent Edmundson–Zagreb measles vaccine has been developed in Yugoslavia that overcomes much of the maternal antibody problem. Field trials at both 6 and 9 months of age have been successful in several developing countries and resulted in seroconversion rates that are equivalent to those of the standard vaccines at 9 and 15 months. Other improved measles vaccines, such as the AIK-C strain developed in Japan, offer equal promise in the future for use in the presence of maternal antibody. It is likely that use of these new vaccines at 6 or 9 months will replace the current vaccine and age at administration (12 months) of the EPI, at least in areas where measles poses a major problem under 1 year of age. Unfortunately, some late increase in mortality has been noted in children receiving these high-potency vaccines (Garenne *et al.*, 1991).

In *developed* countries, the needs are: (1) reaching inner-city children, (2) administration of the vaccine at 9 or 12 months in high-risk groups, such as babies of immigrants from developing countries and low socioeconomic groups (although the Edmundson–Zagreb vaccine is not yet licensed in the United States and we have no high-potency equivalent vaccine), and (3) more intensive vaccination of young adults either who were missed the first time around or who failed to respond to the first injection.

In the United States, the new approach involves vaccination at 9 months in high-risk areas, intensive efforts to reach inner-city populations, and the requirement of a second dose. The Centers for Disease Control Advisory Committee recommends this second dose at the time of entry into grammar school, since other vaccines will be obligatory for school entry in most states. The pediatric advisory group (the Red Book) recommends the second shot at the time of entry into high school. Since a coverage rate of over 98% will be needed to control the spread of measles due to its high infectivity, I feel that a second vaccination at both periods will be needed for several years and until serological surveys validate the fact that an extremely high level of herd immunity has been achieved. About 95% of persons who did not respond to the first injection are said to do so when revaccinated, and further evidence is appearing to document this.

Several new *Haemophilus influenzae* type B (HIB) vaccines, some of them conjugated, have been tested in Finland and in the United States and found to be effective in children over 18 months of age; under that age, where much disease still occurs, the vaccine was not sufficiently immunogenic until a recent study of a conjugated vaccine indicated sufficient evidence to merit licensure. These vaccines are also important in day-care centers and other closed environments where *H. influenzae* poses a significant risk, as well as in developing countries where pneumonia due to this cause results in significant morbidity and mortality. Incorporation of this vaccine and of HBV into the routine EPI program will be desirable in the future. HIB vaccine may even be useful in certain institutional settings for the elderly, where waning childhood immunity is leading to outbreaks of *H. influenzae* infections.

Encouraging results with killed and live cholera and typhoid vaccines are being reported, although the degree and duration of protection for cholera vaccines remain limited. Several attenuated or acellular pertussis vaccines are under development. The question of whether such vaccines will, in rare circumstances, result in late CNS side effects may be epidemiologically unanswerable because of the very large number of persons who must be kept under surveillance, and the occurrence of other causes of CNS diseases. The need for pertussis vaccine in developing countries is clear, however. It is also evident that in developed countries like England, which discontinued vaccine because of concern for reactions, pertussis disease reemerged to a level requiring reinstitution of the vaccine. In general, the cost–benefit ratio would seem to outweigh the risk of complications in developed countries, as it clearly does in developing countries. There is the hope that better vaccines, perhaps molecularly engineered preparations, will emerge that will stimulate the elusive antibody that protects us against infection.

The possibility that new types of time-release adjuvants, such as bio-degradable polymers, can periodically release their antigens at defined intervals over a long period of time, thus eliminating the need for repeated injections, is on the horizon. Such preparations have been successfully used for certain animal vaccines and medications. Vigorous encouragement of this research development is needed, as well as better schedules for more effective delivery of current EPI vaccines. The concept should be promoted in developing countries that vaccination of children be carried out at every contact with the health system, whether they are sick or well, and even at any encounter with governmental agencies, such as nutrition or welfare contacts.

As mentioned earlier, several trials of bovine and monkey derived rotavirus vaccines are under way but have had limited success because of the antigenic diversity of rotavirus strains. A vaccine against HIV is still a remote hope in the eyes of most investigators working on its development. Here, the problems are antigenic diversity, the fact that even natural infection does not produce effective neutralizing antibody, and that the virus destroys the key cells in both humoral and cell-mediated immunity that control most other viral infections. Effective vaccines against respiratory syncytial virus (RSV), gonococcal, chlamydia, syphilis, and malaria infections all seem to be in the more distant future, although molecular tools are providing some key insights into the epitopes that might provide protection. For example, such an epitope has been identified in *B. burgdorferi,* the organism that causes Lyme disease, and trials of a vaccine based on this have been promising in an experimental model.

Our main practical problems today are getting the effective vaccines that are available into the populations that need them. For measles, this means either vaccination in the window of time after the disappearance of maternal antibody and before natural exposure occurs, or the use of vaccines powerful enough to overcome maternal antibody, or by a route, such as intranasal, where humoral antibody would not prevent multiplication of live vaccine in the oral mucosa.

It is not only children who need vaccination, but also the elderly, whose waning immunity and increased exposure in nursing homes are creating problems with infections. In such groups, use of tetanus, influenza, pneumococcal, and perhaps HBV vaccines is far below the level of what we can, and should, attain. In this older age group, antibody levels are dropping from childhood vaccines or natural infections, to which they were exposed earlier in life, so that childhood infections and reactivated viral and bacterial infections are of increasing importance to our senior citizens, who are growing both in numbers and in their life span. This problem is confounded by the close and often unsanitary environment in many of our homes for the elderly, much like some of our day-care nurseries. Respiratory infections such as influenza, *H. influenzae,* tuberculosis, and respiratory syncytial virus, enteric infections such as hepatitis, and recurrent infections such as herpes simplex and herpes zoster viruses are in the high-risk group for these populations. Care of the elderly and of AIDS patients will compete for our health budget. It will be a difficult ethical dilemma, since neither group can be expected to be financially contributing members of society, even after our best medical care is rendered. And for both, life expectancy is limited. With so many poor and uninsured in need of health care, the appropriate way to spend our health dollars poses a critical moral dilemma.

Emergence of New Viruses and New Viral Infections

What new agents can we expect in the future? Several levels in the emergence of new viruses and their subsequent involvement of humans are shown in Table 8.5. I wish to explore some of these levels in more detail, as derived from recent presentations (Evans and Shope, 1989; Evans; 1990). Kilbourne (1990) has also prepared an excellent summary on the challenges of new viral diseases, as presented at a NIH conference, May 2–3, 1989.

The evolution of agents in nature usually involves one or more genetic changes in the virus as it passes through human, animal, or avian hosts. These are depicted in Table 8.6 and include mutation, recombination of animal/avian

Table 8.5
Levels in the Emergence of Viruses and of Host–Virus Interactions

Level
 1 Agent evolving in nature
 2 Agent has evolved but effective human contact has not yet occurred
 3 Effective exposure, infection, and a new disease occurs (new agent, new disease)
 4 Previously latent or nonpathogenic agent produces disease in compromised host (old agent, new disease)
 5 Known viruses in search of diseases or known diseases in search of viruses or the accidental tourist: unknown viruses in search of unknown diseases

Table 8.6
Factors Bearing on Viral Evolution

Viral mutation
  From human passage of virus or in animals by zoonotic agent
Viral recombination
  Recombinants involving human, animal, and avian viruses
Genotypic variation
  Arising from passage in normal or immunocompromised hosts
Emergence of new viral properties
  Genetic alterations affecting virulence, transmission, tissue tropisms, etc.
New animal viruses
  Retroviral infection of nonhuman primates may lead to emergence of latent
  viruses capable of infecting humans
Interspecies infection
  Viruses nonpathogenic for one species may be pathogenic for another
  species

---

strains with human strains, as in influenza, and the emergence of genotypic variants during multiplication in human or animal hosts. Examples of this are HIV, poliovirus, EBV, and other herpesviruses.

Certain general concepts involved in the geographic and transport factors of newly emerged agents are given in Table 8.7. The umbrella concept of malaria hiding many other diseases, as promoted by my associate, the late Dr. Wilbur Downs at Yale, is an important one to remember. In an endemic area, malaria

Table 8.7
Geographic and Transport Factors: General Concepts

---

1. Viruses may evolve *in situ* in isolated and focal geographic areas and be
    transported to human communities by human migration, arthropod
    vectors, animals, or birds.
2. Viruses evolving in indigenous hosts often cause inapparent infection.
3. When viruses are transported to new ecosystems, new geographic areas,
    or new hosts, they often emerge as "new diseases."
4. In order to emerge, viruses need receptive soil, appropriate transport
    mechanisms, and a nonimmune host.
5. Remember "The umbrella of malaria"—many new diseases and viruses
    may hide beneath it.
6. Seek new diseases within old clinical syndromes.

---

parasites are commonly present in the blood of both healthy and diseased persons, so that persons with a febrile illness are often passed off with a diagnosis of malaria when many other infections may be the real cause of the illness. "Challenge the diagnosis," says Dr. Downs, and this is good advice for practitioners of both human and veterinary medicine (Evans, 1990).

Several factors that result in human exposure to new or preexisting agents are listed in Table 8.8. All involve movement of some type: (1) that of the human host to new sites where the agent is present, (2) the movement of the infectious agent by human, animal, avian, insect carriers, or even tissues or cells from these hosts, to a susceptible population, and (3) the introduction of agents into portals of entry in humans that were not previously involved with that agent. New invasive diagnostic procedures, organ transplants, or unusual sexual practices are examples of this.

Table 8.9 presents examples of new or recrudescent viral diseases and some of the risk factors that led to their emergence. Exposure to infected animals, or the introduction of a new vector into the environment, are major reasons for their appearance. In the United States, the importation of the *Aedes albopictus* mosquito into Houston, Texas in old tires imported from Asia, poses the threat of the spread of dengue by this aggressive new vector. In Africa, yellow fever has emerged in several areas. In Nigeria, it occurred as a result of a sylvan outbreak, infection of tourists, and carriage by them to other areas where home water tanks provided a breeding place for the transmitting mosquito. Indeed, the increasing number of tourists in remote areas of the world threatens to become a major human vector for the transmission of infections into their homelands.

Table 8.8
Factors Favoring Effective Contact between Humans and a New
or Preexisting Viral Agent

Factor	Examples
Travel and space exploration	Tropics, ocean depths, archaeological diggings
Human movement	Migration from remote rural to urban settings
Animal movement	Migration or transport into new ecosystems and into new susceptibles
Arthropod or other movement	Either alone or via birds, other vectors, or carriage by airplanes, food, humans
Organ transplants	From other humans or from animals
New portals of entry	New or old agents introduced by new routes, by sexual practices, or by invasive medical procedures

Table 8.9
Examples of New or Recrudescent Viral Diseases

Disease	Area (year)	Risk factors
AIDS	USA (1981→)	Introduction of HIV Homosexual and I.V. spread
Arg. hemorrhagic fever	Argentina (1973)	Rodent exposure Maize harvesting
Bol. hemorrhagic fever	Bolivia (1964, 1971)	Rodent exposure in houses
Ebola fever	Zaire and Sudan (1976)	Patient contact Needle spread
Epidemic polyarthritis	Pacific area	Mosquito-borne
Lassa fever	Nigeria (1969, 1989) Liberia, Sierra Leone (1970–1974)	Hospital exposure Rodent exposure
Marburg disease	Germany (1967) Yugoslavia South Africa (1975)	Exposure to monkey kidney cultures
Rift Valley fever	Egypt (1977)	Local outbreaks, wind, mosquitoes, camels
Yellow fever	Nigeria (1979–1980)	Sylvan yellow fever outbreak Viremic tourists Home water storage

In addition to emergence of new infectious agents in nature, our immunosuppressive drugs may lead to reactivation of old and perhaps previously unrecognized latent pathogenic agents. The appearance of such infections in patients with AIDS is a distressing and epidemic example of this phenomenon and includes viral, bacterial, and parasitic infections. Even rare slow viral infections, such as progressive multifocal leukoencephalopathy, are emerging in AIDS patients with increasing frequency, being reactivated from latent sites in the kidney and then carried to the brain by infected lymphocytes (Chaisson *et al.*, 1990).

In addition, our improving technology and curiosity are discovering new agents in old syndromes. *Legionella pneumophilia* and the new TWAR (Taiwan acute respiratory) chlamydial agents are newly recognized causes of pneumonia. Old agents, or agents previously regarded as nonpathogenic, are producing new syndromes. A historic example is that of *Giardia lamblia*, which was probably the parasite that Leeuwenhoek found in his own stool when he discovered the medical use of the microscope, and which was long believed to be non-pathogenic. Today, it is well known as a widely distributed parasite that causes prolonged diarrhea and weight loss in the unwary traveler or the mountain climber. Parvo virus, type B8, is now recognized as the cause of erythema infectiosum, a common exanthem with a striking lacelike rash occurring in school children. New syndromes of bacterial infection, or of unknown cause, are shown in Table 8.10. Lyme disease, *Legionella* infections, toxic shock, and Kawasaki syndrome are examples of this.

Table 8.11 indicates a number of diseases in which a viral etiology is possible, either as a direct cause, or indirectly, through initiation of an aberrant immune response. Also indicated are those common clinical syndromes in which over half of the causal agents are as yet unknown.

Early Diagnosis and Detection

Given the existence of new agents and the possibility of their involvement with human populations, how shall we set up systems for their early detection? Some suggestions are offered in Table 8.12. Similar, early detection and sentinel systems are important in recognizing new or emerging infectious agents in animals. Veterinarians must work closely with those detecting human infections (Evans, 1990). Indeed, combined units are desirable because most of the new human infections are likely to emerge from animals or birds, or to have counterpart infections in those species. A mobile, internationally staffed expert group under an agency like WHO or CDC with an epidemiology and laboratory unit, or fixed units at critical interfaces between high-risk borders, such as those between the forests of Africa and human habitation, are strongly recommended in an effort to monitor and identify new animal and human infections before they are

Table 8.10
Recent New Bacterial Diseases or of Unknown Cause

Disease factors	Etiology	Possible risk factors
Chronic fatigue syndrome	Unknown	Stress, depression, EBV (?)
Kawasaki disease	Unknown	Rug shampoo, swamps
Legionnaire's disease	*L. pneumophilia*	Cooling towers, smoking
Lyme disease	*B. burgdorferi*	Exposure to infected ticks
Toxic shock	*Staphylococci*	Highly absorbent tampons

Table 8.11
Possible New Virus–Host Interactions: Diseases and Syndromes
with a Possible Viral Etiology

Disease	Possible candidates
Alzheimer's disease	Slow virus?
Insulin-dependent diabetes	Coxsackie B?
Kawasaki disease	Super antigen?
Multiple sclerosis	HTLV-I?
Rheumatoid arthritis	EBV?
Sarcoidosis	?
Systemic lupus erythematosis	?

Common clinical syndromes	Known causes	% Unknown
Central nervous system		
Aseptic meningitis	Enterovirus mumps	80
Encephalitis	HSV, CE, SLE, EE, WE	80
Respiratory system		
Common cold	Rhinovirus, corona	50
Tonsillitis/pharyngitis	HSV, influenza, strepococcus	30
Acute pneumonitis	RSV, parafluenza, *M. pneumoniae*	50
Gastrointestinal system	Rotavirus, Norwalk virus	40

Table 8.12
Early Detection of New Viruses and New Diseases

1. Establish sentinel surveillance and serological units in high-risk areas for emerging viruses supported, if possible, by a high-level laboratory or at least a rapid transport system to one. Monitor and collect blood and other secretions from febrile illnesses.
2. Prepare a mobile team and laboratory under the CDC or WHO, staffed by highly trained microbiologists, epidemiologists, etymologists, etc., that is prepared to leave on a moment's notice to investigate an outbreak of disease anywhere in the world.
3. Set up a "red alert" reporting system for hospital, especially in high-risk areas to report unusual cases or epidemics.

dispersed widely. Possibly, Lassa fever, Marburg disease, Hanta virus, Rift Valley fever, HIV and other retroviruses, and emergent areas of yellow fever activity could have been detected earlier had such laboratories been in operation.

Other Challenges in Infectious Disease Epidemiology

Most of this chapter has dealt with the emergence of new agents and of new agent–host interactions, but there are also other important challenges facing us in infectious disease epidemiology, as listed in Table 8.1. Of very high priority is the need for improved systems of surveillance in both developed and developing countries, utilizing the tremendous power that the computer and improved methods of national and international communication bring to this task. In addition, there is an acute need for the training of more epidemiologists, especially for the developing world. These emerging issues in infectious disease epidemiology have been presented elsewhere (Evans, 1989d, 1990; Evans and Brachman, 1986; Shope and Evans, 1989).

Summary

This chapter has attempted to delineate some of the challenges facing human infectious disease epidemiology in the next decade.

In human diseases, HIV infection, AIDS, and other associated retroviral diseases constitute the biggest challenges in infectious disease epidemiology, now and for the foreseeable future. Indeed, AIDS is one of the major problems of our society, which will affect almost all avenues of human endeavor. Other retroviruses such as HTLV-I are also important, and various hepatitis viruses, herpesviruses, Lyme disease, and tuberculosis are also challenges for the next decade. The effective use of current vaccines in our children, especially in developing countries, is one endeavor in which we are making important progress, but it is questionable that any of these infections will be globally eradicated in the next decade, as was smallpox. However, enormous decreases in clinical cases of measles and of poliomyelitis should occur, with their possible elimination as infectious agents in some countries. New agents will emerge, and we must be prepared to recognize them early and institute early control measures. A good surveillance system in both human and veterinary medicine is critical to these ends. The future will bring important new tools in molecular biology, monoclonal antibody, and rapid diagnostic techniques that will improve our understanding of the transmission of infectious agents, their pathogenesis, the virus–host interrelationships, and development of vaccines for their control.

Control of the host's susceptibility and response to infectious agents may become possible by genetic engineering and immunologic manipulation.

References

Abe J, Kotzen BL, Kazuhito J, *et al:* Selective expansion of T cells expressing T-cell receptor variable B*B*2 and B*B*8 in Kawasaki disease. *Proc Natl Acad Sci USA* **89:**4066–4070, 1992.

Berger, JR, Kaszoity B, Post JD, *et al:* Progressive multifocal leukoencephalopathy associated with human immunodeficiency virus infection: A review of the literature with a report of sixteen cases. *Am Int Med* **107:**78–97, 1987.

Brown P, Goldfarb LV, Gajdusek C: The new biology of spongioform encephalopathy: Infectious amyloidosis with a genetic twist. *Lancet* **1:**1019–1072, 1991.

Centers for Disease Control: First 100,000 cases of acquired immunodeficiency syndrome—United States. *MMWR* **38:**361–363, 1989.

Centers for Disease Control: HIV/AIDS. The first ten years. *MMWR* **40:**357, 1991.

Centers for Disease Control: The second 100,000 cases of acquired immunodeficiency syndrome— United States, June 1981–December 1991. *MMWR* **41:**28–29, 1992.

Chaisson RE, Griffin E: Progressive multifocal leukoencephalopathy in AIDS. *JAMA* **264:**79–82, 1990.

Duesberg P: Retroviruses as carcinogens and pathogens. Expectations and reality. *Cancer Res* **47:**1199–1226, 1987.

Duesberg P: HIV is not the cause of AIDS. *Science* **241:**514–516, 1988.

Evans AS: The need for serological evaluation of immunization programs. *Am J Epidemiol* **112:**735-731, 1980.

Evans AS: Criteria for assessing accomplishments of poliomyelitis control. *Rev Infect Dis* **6**(suppl 2):S5571–S5576, 1984a.

Evans AS: Criteria for the control of infectious diseases using poliomyelitis as an example, *Prog Med Virol* **29:**141–165, 1984b.

Evans AS: The eradication of infectious diseases. Myth or reality? *Am J Epidemiol* **122:**199–207, 1984c.

Evans AS: Ruminations on infectious disease epidemiology: Retrospective, curspective, and prospective. *Int J Epidemiol* **14:**205–211, 1985b.

Evans AS: Subclinical epidemiology. The First Harry A. Feldman Memorial Lecture. *Am J Epidemiol* **125:**545–555, 1987.

Evans AS: The multiple benefits of an AIDS control program. *J AIDS* **1:**415, 1988.

Evans AS: Does HIV cause AIDS? An historical perspective. *J AIDS* **2:**107–113, 1989a.

Evans AS: Etiologic considerations from the epidemiologic picture, in Proceedings of the Third International Congress on Kawasaki Disease, Tokyo, November 29–December 2, 1989b, pp 52–53.

Evans AS: Etiology, in Proceedings of the Third International Congress on Kawasaki Disease, Tokyo, November 29–December 2, 1989c, pp 105–108.

Evans AS: Thoughts on the future of infectious disease epidemiology. Presented at the International Scientific Conference on Epidemiology, April 24–26, 1989d, Beijing, China.

Evans AS: Challenges to the epidemiology of infectious diseases in the next decade, in Adams G., (ed): *Advances in Brucellosis Research.* College Station, Texas A & M University Press, 1990, pp. 321–337.

Evans AS: The chronic fatigue syndrome. Thoughts on pathogenesis. *Rev Infect Dis* **13**(suppl 1):S56–S59, 1991.

Evans AS, Brachman PS: Emerging issues in infectious disease epidemiology. *J Chronic Dis* **39:**1105–1124, 1986.

Evans AS, Mueller N: Viruses and cancer: Causal associations. *Ann Epidemiol* **1:**71–92, 1990.

Gajdusek, C: Slow viral infections. Presented at International Congress on Infectious Diseases, Montreal, Canada, July 15–19, 1990.

Garenne M, Leroy O, Blau JP, *et al:* Child mortality after high titer measles vaccines. Prospective study in Senegal. *Lancet,* **2:**903–907, 1991.

Gold D, Bowden R, Sixby J, *et al:* Chronic fatigue. *JAMA* **264:**48–53, 1990.

Kilbourne E: New viral diseases. *JAMA* **264:**68–70, 1990.

Mann JM: AIDS—The second decade: A global perspective. *J Infect Dis* **165:**245–250, 1992.

Mueller N, Evans A, Harris NL, *et al:* Hodgkin's disease and Epstein–Barr virus: Altered antibody pattern before diagnosis. *N Engl J Med* **320:**689–695, 1989.

Mueller N, Evans AS, *et al:* Non-Hodgkin's lymphoma and EBV: Evidence of altered virus activity prior to diagnosis (in press).

National Institute of Allergy and Infectious Diseases: Program for accelerated development of new vaccines. 1985 Progress Report. Bethesda, NIH, 1985.

Purtillo, D, Luka J, Patton D, *et al:* EBV genome detection in Kawasaki disease. Presented at the Fifth International Symposium on Epstein-Barr virus and associated diseases, Annency, France, Sept. 13–19, 1992, Abstract No P-VI-32, p 160.

Shope R, Evans AS: Assessing geographic factors and transport: Recognition of new factors, in: Morse SS (ed), *Emerging Viruses.* New York, Oxford University Press, 1993, pp 109–119.

Stoeckel P, Schlumberger G, Parent B, *et al:* Use of killed poliovirus vaccine in a routine immunization program in West Africa. *Rev Infect Dis* **6**(suppl 2):S463–S467, 1984.

Zur Hausen H: Viruses in human cancer. *Science* **254:**1173–1187, 1991.

Causation and Chronic Diseases

While the same general epidemiological principles apply to both acute (infec-tious) and chronic (noninfectious) diseases, there are many differences that pro-foundly affect the ease of establishing causal inferences. Indeed, the complexity is such in chronic diseases that the term "risk factor" rather than "cause" is usually applied. It should be emphasized that while the term "noninfectious" is applied to chronic disease, it is more accurate to say noncontagious, because some infectious agents are causally related to a chronic or malignant disease. These include chronic diseases of the central nervous system due to viruses (see Chapter 4), several malignant diseases as reviewed in Chapter 5, and a number of chronic conditions of suspected viral etiology such as juvenile, insulin-dependent diabetes, rheumatoid arthritis, and systemic lupus erythematosis. Acquired im-munodeficiency disease (AIDS) also fits this category. These latter diseases are reviewed in terms of establishing their infectious etiologies in a fine paper by Norden and Kuller (1984). Traditional infectious diseases may also pursue a long-term, chronic course such as tuberculosis, syphilis, Lyme disease, and AIDS, to mention a few.

The major differences between infectious diseases and true noninfectious disease epidemiology are listed in Table 9.1, as derived from papers by Lilienfeld (1973) and Kuller (1987). The inability to isolate and replicate an agent in the laboratory and to reproduce the disease in an experimental animal are major obstacles to fulfilling the Henle–Koch postulates. The absence of an immune response invalidates Rivers's and Huebner's criterion of proof in viral diseases. The long incubation period of most chronic diseases and the inability to ascertain the exact risk factors present at the time when the pathological process began are confounded by the multiple cofactors involved in the pathogenesis of most chronic diseases. While inapparent infections are typical of most infectious agents, and can be identified by isolation of the agent and/or demonstration of an immune response, such subclinical processes undoubtedly occur in many true

Table 9.1
Some Comparisons between Infectious and Chronic Disease Epidemiology[a]

Characteristic	Infectious disease	Chronic disease
Agent	Replicates	Does not replicate
Can be grown in lab?	Yes, for most agents	No
Can be reproduced in animals?	Yes, for many agents	No, with some exceptions (certain toxins, carcinogens)
Induce immunity?	Yes, except HIV	No immune response
Incubation period	Usually short and defined (except long with kuru and AIDS)	Usually long and indefinite
Epidemics	Common and often of short duration (except for AIDS)	Occur for some diseases over a long period (lung cancer, coronary heart disease)
Contagiousness?	Yes, but variable for most agents	Not in true sense, but behavioral spread occurs
Subclinical cases	Very common for most infections	May occur if laboratory markers are available
Multiple causes or risk factors	Infectious agent necessary but cofactors involved in appearance of disease	Common and complicated in a "web of causation"

[a]From Lilienfeld (1973) and Kuller (1987).

chronic diseases, as reviewed in Chapter 12. For some of these diseases, there are good laboratory markers of the existence of this subclinical pathological process.

In this chapter, the focus will be on more classical chronic diseases of a noninfectious origin (as far as we know) and on the development of criteria or guidelines to establish causal inferences. The following discussion is derived, sometimes verbatim, from a previous article on this topic (Evans, 1976).

The impetus for criteria that apply to causation in chronic diseases came largely from recognition of the association of smoking and lung cancer in 1950 (Wynder and Graham, 1950) and later the recognition that cholesterol (as well as smoking and obesity) played a role in the development of coronary artery disease, as shown in the great Framingham study (Thomas *et al.*, 1966). Keys's (1970) study of dietary habits in seven countries and the relation of diet and heart disease indicated that many geographic factors were involved in this process. An early effort to establish some guidelines regarding causal inferences from such associations was a conference held in 1958 where Jakob Yerushalmy (Figure 9.1) and Palmer developed a set of criteria (Yerushalmy and Palmer, 1959). First, they reviewed Koch's postulates and stressed that, in relation to their possible application to chronic disease, two essential types of evidence were (1) the simultaneous presence of the organism and the disease and their appearance in the correct sequence and (2) the specificity of the effect of the organism on the development of the disease. In particular, the need was stressed to establish the *specificity* of an effect in studies of chronic diseases. The concept of multiple causation was also emphasized in chronic diseases as opposed to acute infectious diseases.

In applying the criteria, three problems were mentioned: (1) the difficulty of measurement, (2) the selection of controls against whom an increase in frequency may be gauged, and (3) the question of the correct sequence of events. Table 9.2 presents their guidelines (Yerushalmy and Palmer, 1959). The first two guidelines reflected their derivation from Koch's first two postulates, but the two statements were not to be regarded as independent. Retrospective studies are

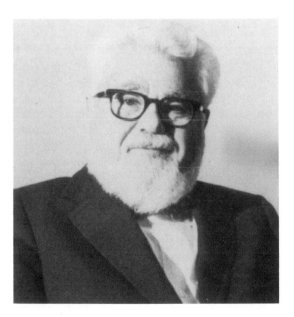

Figure 9.1. Jakob Yerushalmy, 1904–1973, Professor of Biostatistics, University of California, Berkeley (from Evans, 1976).

Table 9.2
**Guideposts for Implication of a Characteristic as an Etiologic Factor
in a Chronic Disease[a]**

1. The suspected characteristic must be found more frequently in persons with the disease in question than in persons without the disease, or
2. Persons possessing the characteristic must develop the disease more frequently than do persons not possessing the characteristic.
3. An observed association between a characteristic and a disease must be tested for validity by investigating the relationship between the characteristics and other diseases and, if possible, the relationship of similar or related characteristics to the disease in question. The suspected characteristic can be said to be specifically related to the disease in question when the results of such investigation indicate that similar relationships do not exist with a variety of characteristics and with many disease entities when such relationships are not predictable on physiologic, pathologic, experimental, or epidemiologic grounds. In general, the lower the frequency of these other associations, the higher is the specificity of the original observed association and the higher the validity of the causal inference.

[a]From Yerushalmy and Palmer (1959).

usually involved in establishing the first guideline and prospective or cohort studies in establishing the second. In their view, it should not be necessary to fulfill both criteria, although the first one does not involve establishing the temporal sequence of the suspected characteristic in relation to the development of the disease—a critical element in causal proof. The authors were most concerned with the proper selection of controls. For example, a comparison between lung cancer in smokers and in nonsmokers was not valid unless other characteristics were shown to be similar in the two groups. This was because some other characteristic of the smoker, other than smoking itself, might be the real risk factor. As an item for discussion at the conference, they presented the third guideline shown in Table 9.2.

Abraham Lilienfeld, shown in Figure 9.2, discussed the presentation. He pointed out that one might consider "vectors" in chronic diseases, just as in infectious diseases, in that cigarette smoke is the "vector" of lung cancer just as polluted water is the vector of typhoid fever and cholera (Lilienfeld, 1959a,b). He indicated that while identification of the *specific* agent present in the "vector" was important, it was not necessary to develop practical methods of control. Just as elimination of exposure to polluted water can control typhoid fever, so the elimination of exposure to cigarette smoke can reduce lung cancer, without the need to identify either the typhoid bacillus in water or the carcinogen in cigarette smoke. In this paper and in other publications (1959a,b; 1966), Lilienfeld made certain modifications in the guidelines of Yerushalmy and Palmer, and these are given in Table 9.3. The interplay of the multiple factors involved in the causation of chronic disease has been termed "the web of causation" in the text by Mac-Mahon *et al.* (1960). Susser has presented a complete discussion of causal thinking, and of ways to establish causation, in his fine book, *Causal Thinking in the Health Sciences* (1973). Many epidemiologists have become involved in issues of causation and of causal inferences (Rothman, 1976; Sartwell, 1960; Holland, 1986; Susser, 1991), and this issue has involved clinicians as well (Bollet, 1964; Feinstein, 1979).

The problem of establishing objective criteria for causation was a direct challenge to the Surgeon General's Advisory Group on Smoking and Health in 1964 (Surgeon General, 1964). They set up a series of attributes that related evidence of association between a suspected cause (smoking) and a disease (lung

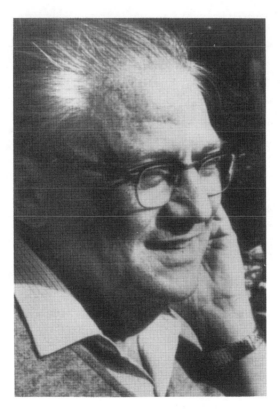

Figure 9.2. Abraham M. Lilienfeld, 1920–1985, Professor of Epidemiology, School of Hygiene and Public Health, Johns Hopkins University (from Evans, 1976).

Table 9.3
Added Criteria in Establishing Causation in Chronic Disease[a]

1. The incidence of the disease should increase in relation to the duration and intensity (dose) of the suspected factor.
2. The distribution of the suspected factor should parallel that of the disease in all relevant aspects.
3. A spectrum of illness should be related to exposure to the suspected factor.
4. Reduction or removal of the factor should reduce or stop the disease.
5. Human populations exposed to the factor in controlled studies should develop the disease more commonly than those not so exposed.

[a]Based on Lilienfeld (1957, 1959a,b, 1966).

cancer), as summarized in Table 9.4. Similar criteria were published by Bradford Hill in relation to occupational cancer at about the same time (1965) and are discussed in detail in Chapter 10, as well as in a recent paper by Susser (1991).

Toward a Unified Concept

There are a number of limitations that the investigator seeking causal inferences from data in either acute or chronic disease should recognize, and are in addition to the web of defined risk factors that appear to be involved in the pathogenesis of a disease in a given setting or population group. These are: (1) the same pathological or clinical condition can result from different sets of risk factors in different settings. (2) The risk factors may vary in different geographic areas, in different age groups, in different behavioral groups, and in different patterns of host susceptibility, particularly genetic (Evans, 1967). The extent to which a given set of risk factors is responsible in a defined setting for producing a

Table 9.4
Elements of Causation in Chronic Disease[a]

1. The consistency of the association
2. The strength of the association
3. The specificity of the association
4. The temporal relationship of the association
5. The coherence of the association.

[a]From Surgeon General (1964).

clinical disease has been termed "attributable risk." It is a measure to identify the proportion of a specific disease associated with a given cause (Levin, 1953; Lilienfeld, 1973). Thus, abstention from smoking might reduce the incidence of lung cancer by some 70%, other factors being constant, just as an effective vaccine against the rhinoviruses might reduce the incidence of the common cold by some 25%. (3) Most diseases, including infectious diseases, require the presence of several risk factors (multiple causation) before clinical disease develops (see Chapter 11); the variability of the host response on exposure to these same risk factors is enormous, mostly for ill-defined or unknown reasons. (4) A single strong risk factor or infectious agent may produce different clinical and pathological responses under different circumstances. For example, *Chlamydia trachomatis* can result in a broad spectrum of different clinical responses involving the eye, lung, or genital tract, just as smoking may lead to a variety of chronic conditions from heart disease to emphysema to bladder cancer. (5) In addition to these qualitative differences in response patterns, any cause or set of causes (or risk factors) can result in a quantitative spectrum of host response ranging from inapparent or subclinical illness to severe and fatal disease.

A causative agent or risk factor of low pathogenicity or low potency may be able to induce clinical disease only in human hosts rendered more susceptible by exposure at a given age, or when the immune system or some other protective mechanism is impaired, or in the presence of a cofactor. Thus, the whole spectrum of infectious and malignant conditions appearing in persons infected with HIV is the result of destruction of CD4 T lymphocytes involved in defense against infectious agents and malignant cells. Advances in molecular biology and in genetics are providing increasing insight into the effect of molecular changes in the agent and in genetic attributes of the host on the agent–host interaction. Genes are being identified and cloned that result in susceptibility to certain chronic diseases such as Alzheimer's disease and in resistance, such as the repressor gene for retinoblastoma. Mutations in gene p53 may be a more generic marker of susceptibility. When exposure to a risk factor is very widespread, such as herpesvirus or HIV in infectious diseases, or fat or smoking in chronic diseases, it may be very difficult to prevent exposure, and if not possible to do so, identification and modification of host response patterns based on newer molecular and genetic knowledge will become increasingly important.

The common features of these considerations of causation for both acute and chronic diseases have encouraged me to develop a working set of criteria for causation, or "unified concept," as presented in Table 9.5. This represents a generic guideline for practical guidance in seeking whether a given characteristic represents merely an association or is a true causal or risk factor for the disease or that proportion attributable to it. They have been slightly modified by Black and Lilienfeld (1984) as guidelines to causation in legal tort cases. These criteria have also been included as "Evans's postulates" in Last's *A Dictionary of Epi-*

Table 9.5
Criteria for Causation: A Unified Concept[a]

1. *Prevalence* of the disease should be significantly higher in those exposed to the putative cause than in matched controls not so exposed.[b]
2. *Exposure* to the putative cause should be present more commonly in those with the disease than in controls without the disease when all risk factors are held constant.
3. *Incidence* of the disease should be significantly higher in those exposed to the putative cause than in those not so exposed as shown in prospective studies.
4. *Temporally*, the disease should *follow* exposure to the putative agent with a distribution of incubation periods on a bell-shaped curve.
5. A *spectrum* of host responses should follow exposure to the putative agent along a logical biologic gradient from mild to severe.
6. A *measurable host response* following exposure to the putative cause should *regularly appear* in those lacking this before exposure (i.e., antibody, cancer cells) or should *increase* in magnitude if present before exposure; this pattern should not occur in persons not so exposed.
7. *Experimental reproduction* of the disease should occur in higher incidence in animals or man appropriately exposed to the putative cause than in those not so exposed; this exposure may be deliberate in volunteers, experimentally induced in the laboratory, or demonstrated in a controlled regulation of natural exposure.
8. *Elimination or modification* of the putative cause or of the vector carrying it should decrease the incidence of the disease (control of polluted water or smoke or removal of the specific agent).
9. *Prevention* or *modification* of the host's response on exposure to the putative cause should decrease or eliminate the disease (immunization, drug to lower cholesterol, specific lymphocyte transfer factor in cancer).
10. The whole thing should make biologic and epidemiologic sense.

---

[a]From Evans (1976).
[b]The putative cause may exist in the external environment or in a defect in host response.

demiology (1983), but it should be emphasized that: (1) they are based on the work of others, especially Yerushalmy, Palmer, and Lilienfeld, (2) they are subject to change, as new technology, particularly new molecular and genetic techniques, are applied to causation, and as new concepts of pathogenesis and susceptibility appear. Furthermore, they must be modified to meet the special needs of specific diseases in which restriction in methods limits their application, such as slow viral diseases and immunological diseases, and (3) they are epidemiological in nature rather than molecular, such as criteria for the relationship of viruses to cancer (Zur Hausen, 1991).

References

Black B, Lilienfeld DE: Epidemiologic proof in toxic tort litigation. *Fordham U Law Rev* **52:**723–785, 1984.

Bollet AJ: On seeking the cause of a disease. *Clin Res* **12:**305–310, 1964.

Evans AS: Causation and disease: The Henle–Koch postulates revisited. *Yale J Biol Med* **49:**175–195, 1976.

Feinstein AR: Clinical biostatistics. 48. Efficacy of different research structures in preventing bias in the analysis of causation. *Clin Pharmacol Ther* **26:**129–141, 1979.

Hill AB: The environment and disease: Association or causation? *Proc R Soc Med* **58:**295–300, 1965.

Holland PW: Statistics and causal inference. *J Am Stat Assoc* **81:**945–960, 1986.

Keys A (ed): Coronary heart disease in seven countries. *Circulation* suppl 1, 1970.

Kuller LH: Relationship between acute and chronic disease epidemiology. *Yale J Biol Med* **60:**363–376, 1987.

Last JM: *A Dictionary of Epidemiology.* London, Oxford University Press, 1983.

Levin ML, Goldstein H, Gerhardt, PR: Cancer and tobacco smoking. *JAMA* **143:**336–338, 1950.

Lilienfeld A: Epidemiological methods and inferences in studies of non-infectious disease. *Public Health Rep* **72:**51–60, 1959a.

Lilienfeld AM: On the methodology of investigations of etiologic factors in chronic disease—Some comments. *J Chronic Dis* **10:**41–46, 1959b.

Lilienfeld AM: Epidemiologic methods and inferences, in Lilienfeld AM, Gifford AJ (eds): *Chronic Diseases and Public Health.* Baltimore, Johns Hopkins University Press, 1966.

Lilienfeld AM: Epidemiology of infectious and non-infectious disease. Some comparisons. *Am J Epidemiol* **97:**135–147, 1973.

MacMahon B, Pugh TF, Ipsen J: *Epidemiologic Methods.* Boston, Little Brown & Co, 1960.

Norden CW, Kuller LH: Identifying infectious etiologies of chronic disease. *Rev Infect Dis* **6:**200–213, 1984.

Rothman KJ: Causes. *Am J Epidemiol* **104:**587–592, 1976.

Sartwell PE: On the methodology of investigation of etiologic factors in chronic diseases—Further comments. *J Chronic Dis* **11:**61–63, 1960.

Surgeon General, Advisory Committee of the U.S.P.H.S., "Smoking and Health," PHS Publ No. 1103. Washington, DC, Superintendent of Documents, 1964.

Susser M: *Causal Thinking in the Health Sciences: Concepts and Strategies in Epidemiology.* London, Oxford University Press, 1973.

Susser M: What is a cause and how do we know one? A grammar for pragmatic epidemiology. *Am J Epidemiol* **133:**635–648, 1991.

Thomas EH Jr, Kannel WB, Dawber TR, *et al:* Cholesterol in phosphorylated ratio in the prediction of coronary heart disease. The Framingham study. *N Engl J Med* **274:**701–705, 1966.

Wynder EL, Graham EA: Tobacco smoking as a possible etiologic factor in bronchogenic carcinoma. *JAMA* **143:**329–336, 1950.

Yerushalmy J, Palmer CE: On the methods of investigations of etiologic factors in chronic diseases. *J Chronic Dis* **18:** 27–40, 1959.

Zur Hausen H: Papilloma/host cell interactions in the pathogenesis of anorectal cancer, in: *Origins of Cancer: A Comprehensive Review.* Cold Spring Harbor, New York, Cold Spring Harbor Lab Press, 1991, pp 685–688.

10

Causation and Occupational Diseases

Introduction

The proof that an occupational or environmental exposure produces a particular disease involves not only scientific and epidemiological evidence, but also the legal aspects of proof. These include "cause in fact" and "proximate cause." The court must also decide who is liable for the exposure, the degree to which the exposure accounted for the disease, and the amount of financial compensation due the plaintiff. Medical malpractice suits are another type of legal problem in causation. In addition to the individual toxic tort case, there are other types of legal cases in which causation must be evaluated such as environmental exposures arising from industry, toxic wastes, nuclear plants, aerosol spraying, and other sources in which groups of persons are exposed. The defendant in such cases may be an industry, a municipality, the armed forces, or the government itself. There are also widespread legal issues involved in consumer suits for presumed reactions or diseases resulting from food additives, drugs, and vaccines.

This chapter will focus primarily on causation in toxic tort cases resulting in chronic or malignant diseases. The acute exposure and the accidental injury will be excluded from this discussion because causation is generally more apparent, and because these cases are usually settled through the Workmen's Compensation Act with their own investigators. The time period between exposure and the presumed effect is usually short. There are exceptions to this in which the incubation period is long and the causal relationship less obvious. These fall into the area to be discussed in this chapter where the nature, dosage, and duration of the exposure are critical elements and in which there may be several types of resulting diseases. There are both epidemiological and legal problems in establishing causation in toxic tort cases and each will be discussed separately.

177

Epidemiological Issues

The difficulties of establishing causality in most occupational diseases are similar to those encountered in the malignant and chronic diseases occurring outside industry that have already been discussed in Chapter 5. However, in occupational cases it must be shown that exposure to the presumed causative agent occurred in the workplace because the same disease due to the same or different causes may occur outside the workplace. Indeed, exposure in both the home and workplace may contribute to the same disease and the extent to which each is responsible must be determined in court for purposes of establishing the degree of liability: this is termed "attributable risk." For occupational diseases the *place of exposure,* its *dosage and duration,* and the *time* between first exposure in the workplace and the onset of the disease are critical elements of causation in toxic tort cases in determining "beyond a reasonable doubt" that *that* exposure resulted in *that* disease in *that* individual. These are requirements in specificity far beyond the general criteria for epidemiological proof required in the population groups with which epidemiology generally deals.

General epidemiological principles and specific methodologies to prove causation in occupational exposures have been presented at a recent conference by Leon Gordis (1986) and Mervyn Susser (1986). Several epidemiological methods have been used in identifying possible causal relationships between an occupational exposure and a disease, in finding which industries are more hazardous than others, and in ascertaining which diseases are more common in specific occupations. In identifying hazardous occupations, the mortality or morbidity rates are determined in different industries, as compared with the rates in the general population, or in some more comparable control population. Where an excess is found, then an investigation is begun in an attempt to identify the particular disease or diseases that account for the increase and to search for the possible exposures that may have played a causal role in their pathogenesis. Another approach is to determine the incidence or prevalence rates for specific chronic or malignant diseases in different occupations as compared with some control group. This may consist of unexposed persons, or the general population, or the populations outside the plants who are in that specific regional area. The application of these epidemiological approaches to the proof of specific causal relationships is not easy in these types of case–control studies. The problems in malignant diseases, which apply equally to many chronic diseases, have been well set forth by Sir Richard Doll (Figure 10.1), one of the world's great epidemiologists, in a paper titled "Occupational Cancer: A Hazard for Epidemiologists" (Doll, 1985). He points out the epidemiological data must be used to supplement laboratory tests in the search for occupational carcinogens in order

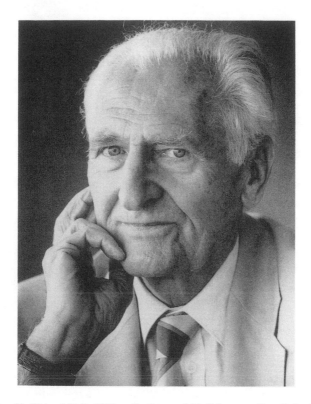

Figure 10.1. Sir Richard Doll, 1912– , Professor of Medicine, emeritus, Oxford University.

"(1) to discover risks that have been overlooked or suggested only tentatively by laboratory tests, (2) to check the correctness of conclusions about monitoring the effect of its removal, and (3) to estimate the level of response that produces the highest additional risk of disease that is socially acceptable." He also emphasizes that epidemiology must be employed not only to show that an agent is carcinogenic but also to show that it is not. The assignment of a clean bill of health to a presumed carcinogen that has been incriminated on inadequate or missing evidence may be difficult but is an important challenge for future epidemiologists. This involves not only establishing the scientific evidence that a substance is harmless but the commitment in published form to this conviction. In my view, societies like the American College of Epidemiology must undertake this difficult ethical and moral task of identifying which exposures are harmful and which are not, using their best judgment. Errors will be made but only expert and informed opinion can lead the way out of the current confusion.

At present, there appear to be 17 agents or groups of agents that are well established by laboratory and epidemiological evidence as having caused cancer in 35 broad occupational groups, as summarized for the International Labour Office by Simonato and Saracci (1983). Doll (1985) states that "No one would, I think, question the validity of the evidence that led to the construction of this list, although they might question whether it was right to describe arsenic, chromium, and nickel as carcinogens, rather than some of their compounds." However, this list should be very useful as a point of reference in occupational cases involving exposure to these carcinogens. There is a second list of agents in which "the assessment of the carcinogenic risk is not definitive" and with which Doll takes some exception. This list is composed of 66 occupational groups in 14 of which the suspected agent is undefined. This list may be helpful in cases involving toxic torts but would require expert evaluation at the time of the trial for each presumed carcinogen. In addition, new suspected or proven carcinogens are being identified all the time. For example, Doll (1985) mentions 8 new types of cancer due to three established occupational carcinogens (asbestos, chromium, and vinyl chloride) and added 17 new types associated with six groups of occupations. Some recent estimates are that 20–30% of all cancers arise from occupational exposures.

The assessment of epidemiological evidence between the occupational exposure and the chronic and malignant diseases that are presumed to result is not easy. Doll has stated it this way: "if there is one general rule, it is that conclusions can not be reached until the totality of the evidence is taken into account; and this not only includes the results of all available occupational studies, but may also include general geographic and temporal trends in incidence (particularly in the case of rare cancers) and will, of course, always include the laboratory evidence as well."

In addition to the case–control studies discussed above, long-term, prospective investigations are being carried out in cohorts of persons exposed to identifiable and specific agents, suspected of being possible causes of chronic or malignant diseases. To their credit, many industries are making such risk assessments and epidemiologists are being increasingly employed in the pursuit of these studies. This approach is costly and time-consuming but if conducted properly with equal follow-up of exposed and nonexposed groups they provide the highest order of a causal relationship next to randomized exposure trials, which are ethically impossible to conduct. Unfortunately, the publication of the results of such investigations, especially if positive, or if they can be construed as positive, provide litigious lawyers with the opportunity for court trials that may adversely affect the industry.

The discussion of specific guidelines or criteria to aid in determining causation in occupational diseases will be delayed in this chapter until some of the special legal elements of causality are presented.

Legal Issues

Most legal issues involve the problems of court trials for diseases presumably resulting from some occupational exposure to a harmful substance or toxin. These cases are called toxic torts. The difficulties have been well reviewed in excellent papers by Harter (1985, 1986) entitled "The Dilemma of Causation in Toxic Torts." He defines toxic torts as "a legal claim for compensation for a disease that is alleged to have resulted from an exposure to some agent for which the defendant is in some way responsible." Another fine paper reviewing these issues and the application of epidemiological principles to toxic tort cases by B. Black, a lawyer, and D. Lilienfeld, an epidemiologist, uses the same concept (1984). Both papers focus on chronic diseases associated with a single exposure and exclude acute illnesses with a short incubation period. The problem was again considered by Black at a conference on causation and financial compensation (1986). The issues of multiple causation and of interaction with other factors are not generally addressed in these papers, nor will they be in this chapter because of the complexity involved.

Workmen's compensation cases are not regarded as torts in the classical sense, although some raise similar questions related to causation, such as a long incubation period between exposure and disease and the intensity and duration of the exposure. This long latent or incubation period between exposure to a presumed toxic substance and the later development of a malignant or chronic disease may often exceed the statute of legal limitations, usually on the order of 4 to 6 years. For example, mesotheliomas due to asbestos (plus cigarette smoking), angiosarcomas after exposure to vinyl chloride, and nasal sinus cancers following working with nickel or its compounds seldom occur less than 15 years after the onset of exposure. However, some occupational cancers occur within 10 years and bladder cancers under 5 years. Some of the incubation periods for certain chronic and malignant diseases for which the time of exposure is relatively certain are listed in Table 10.1 as derived from a paper by Armenian and Lilienfield (1974).

The magnitude of deaths from occupational diseases is generally regarded to be high. Harter (1985) quotes Ashford's estimate, placing it at some 100,000 occupationally related deaths per year. In most of these cases, legal compensation is neither sought nor denied because of the difficulty in proving causation. Other authorities feel that Ashford's estimate is far too high (Weil, 1983) and that the legal recoveries in financial compensation exceed the scientific basis on which the decisions are made due to sympathy for the claimant, a belief in the "deep pockets" of the defendants or the insurers, and a general perception that illnesses resulting from exposure are a major public health problem (Harter, 1986). The financial burden of some of these cases may be immense, especially in occupational or environmental exposures involving many persons such as the

Table 10.1
Estimated Median of the Incubation or Latent Period between Occupational or Environmental Exposures and the Development of Certain Malignant Diseases[a]

Exposure	Disease	No. of cases	Median incubation period (years)
Asbestos	Lung cancer	69	36.5
Atom bomb	Leukemia		
Hiroshima		83	6.8
Nagasaki		36	7.2
Occupational dyes	Bladder cancer		
Series A		100	17.5
Series B		?	16.3
Radiation			
General	Leukemia		
	Ankylosing spondylitis	52	6.4
Thyroid[b]	Adenoma	60	17.8
	Cancer	132	9.6
Intrauterine	Wilms's tumor	41	2.1

[a]Modified from Armenian and Lilienfeld (1974) and Lilienfeld and Lilienfeld (1982).
[b]Thyroid disease in childhood.

Bhopal, India exposure to cyanide gas, the Three Mile Island exposure to radiation, the air pollution from Agent Orange during the Vietnam conflict, and the emanations from toxic wastes at Love Canal. The epidemiological evidence of the validity of some of these claims will be discussed at the end of this chapter.

Another important legal issue in toxic tort compensation in the United States is payment for "pain and suffering," as well as "punitive costs" for liability, which are added to the costs of medical compensation. Also, the reimbursement costs for medical care do not usually take into account other medical insurance or health care plans that the plaintiff may have. These difficult issues in establishing a reasonable scientific and legal basis for causation and for awarding financial compensation were addressed at a 1985 meeting on "Causation and Financial Compensation" sponsored by Georgetown University and which involved lawyers, judges, insurance experts, physicians involved in occupational diseases, and epidemiologists. This meeting, in which this author participated, has been a major stimulus and source of information for this chapter.

The nature of the plaintiff and of the defendant vary greatly in different toxic tort cases. If the exposure arises in the course of a person's work, then suit will usually be against the suppliers of the plaintiff's employers because workmen's compensation statutes usually prohibit employees from suing their employers for injuries and illnesses arising from the workplace (Harter, 1986). If the exposure arises in the environment, then the defendant is the person or company alleged to have produced or released the toxin, or allowed it to be placed or remain in an area where the public is exposed (as in Love Canal). In toxic tort cases involving consumers of a product such as a drug or vaccine, the pharmaceutical houses that manufactured it are being increasingly sued. An example of this is the Cutter incident in which paralytic poliomyelitis resulted from administration of a presumedly killed vaccine but in which some particles escaped inactivation despite the fact that the manufacturer followed the appropriate protocol for its preparation. The problem was later identified as a failure to break up and filter the viral particles so that some in the center of clumps escaped exposure to the formaldehyde used to kill the virus: this phenomenon had not been recognized in the original protocol. Another type of legal issue arises in the case of drugs or vaccines in which there is an inherent risk of side reactions due to the basic nature of the product or to individual susceptibility to some component. The side reactions from pertussis vaccine, for example, have resulted in so many suits that all but one U.S. manufacturer have ceased production. Oral poliomyelitis vaccine may result in paralysis in less than one in a million of those who receive it or who are intimately exposed to persons who receive it. This appears to be an unavoidable risk and society must decide whether this miniscule risk should deter the great and proven benefit of vaccination. In some of these cases the physician administering the vaccine is held accountable for lack of properly informing the patient of the risk involved. This concept of "informed consent" when applied to all of the pharmaceuticals and vaccines used in medical therapy and prophylaxis provides eager lawyers a motive to take on suits on a contingency basis. Greater participation by the government in co-insuring against some of the unavoidable problems where the health of the public is concerned would seem urgent and/or changes in the legal system that limit liability. Other recent medical-legal issues include the development of vaginal cancer in the young adult female children of pregnant women given diethylstilbestrol (DES), gynecological complications resulting from use of the Dalkon shield in contraception, and the appearance of the toxic shock syndrome in menstruating women using certain types of tampons. The government is also now involved in many of these suits; e.g., the occurrence of Guillain–Barre syndrome following the mass government-sponsored immunization program against swine influenza, to be discussed later, and the uses of the defoliant Agent Orange containing dioxin during the Vietnam conflict. In all of these, both medical and legal elements required for establishing causation are involved. The next section will discuss the legal aspects.

Causation and the Law

Causation in legal terms involves two issues: (1) causation in fact and (2) proximate cause. The former can be defined as anything in the chain of events that led to an injury or disease and without which it would not have happened, i.e., it is a necessary causal event (Harter, 1985, 1986). Thus, if an injury or illness would not have occurred without the event (causal factor), it is not a "cause in fact" of that effect. Because this definition is too broad to assign liability, more recent usage has been modified to one that measures the *contribution* of the event to the injury or disease and this must be judged to be a "substantial factor" in bringing about the injury before it will be regarded as a "cause in fact" (Harter, 1985). The question is what *in fact* has occurred. The plaintiff must prove that the conduct of the defendant was a substantial factor in bringing about the result. Thus, proof of causation in law seems to rest both on the role of the causal agent in bringing about the effect and on the defendant whose actions resulted in the particular exposure. Both must be shown to be "substantial factors." The second legal criterion, that of "proximate cause," is a matter of law or policy as to whether to impose liability on someone who is presumably responsible for a "cause in fact" of the injury or illness. This issue usually involves the demonstration that the "cause in fact" increased the risk, and the determination as to whether the disease or injury was a "reasonably foreseeable" result of the defendant's actions. It is the nature of the risk itself and not the possible extent of the damages actually sustained that is involved in what is foreseeable. If the risk was foreseeable, then liability may extend to the full extent of the damages whether they were foreseen or unforeseen.

These two legal concepts of "cause in fact" and "proximate cause" have now been combined in a "Restatement of Torts" into the single term "legal cause." This defines an event as causal if it is a substantial factor in bringing about harm.

Elements of Causal Proof in the Law

Some of the steps, questions, and problems in toxic tort cases are summarized in Table 10.2 and include establishing causation, assigning liability, and determining the amount of financial compensation. To establish causation, the plaintiff must demonstrate "by a preponderance of the evidence" that the defendant's actions were a substantial factor in producing the harm. The plaintiff must present enough evidence to provide a reasonable basis for reasonable people (the jurors) to decide that it is "more likely than not" that the actions were, in fact, a substantial factor in causing the injury or disease. The decision of the "more likely than not" issue is based on a so-called 50+% test (more than a 50% chance that it was the cause). It is a judgmental decision the jury must make on the basis of often conflicting evidence presented by the lawyers or expert witnesses for the plaintiff on the one hand, and those for the defendant on the other. Such adver-

Table 10.2
Basic Questions and Problems in Toxic Tort Cases

1. Can the preponderance of evidence establish that exposure A caused disease B in more than 50% of the cases and can the evidence fulfill scientific postulates of causation (Henle–Koch–Evans)?
2. If the answer to number 1 is yes, then to what extent did that exposure produce the disease over other exposures that can also produce the same disease, i.e., what is the attributable risk to that exposure alone?
3. Was *that particular exposure* "more likely than not" the cause of *that particular disease* in *that particular person*?
4. If the preponderance of evidence supports "causation in fact," then who was responsible for the exposure and was the risk of disease foreseen?
5. If the risk was foreseen, then should the person responsible be held accountable for *all* diseases following exposure?
6. Should the person accountable for the exposure be asked to compensate for (a) all medical costs or just the portion due to the attributable risk concept? (b) Should compensation be limited just to costs over and above other sources of insurance coverage or for all costs? (c) Should compensation be required for "pain and suffering" and for "punitive damages"?
7. Are the legal and administrative costs of establishing "cause in fact" justified given the difficulty of establishing causation on the "more likely than not" principle and when adversarial evidence is presented by lawyers for the plaintiff and the defendants before a judge and jury usually untrained in the scientific grounds for proof?

sarial presentations are likely to emphasize the extremes of the epidemiological and laboratory evidence available, when it is difficult enough for independent and objective specialists in causation to come to valid consensus. In practice, "truth lies in the eyes of the beholder" so that the persuasiveness of the argument presented by the lawyer for either the plaintiff or the defendant may influence the jury as much as the scientific and objective evidence itself. The legal requirement of "more likely than not" is in contrast to the usual medical or epidemiological approach. Here "the most likely cause" is the usual term used as determined by statistical data, relative risk calculations, and the attributable risk of the exposure itself. The implication of the legal definition is not only that it was the most likely cause but that, in fact, it was "more likely than not" *the* cause of the injury or the disease. According to Harter (1985), the law has great difficulty in dealing with "statistical evidence" because of three concerns: (1) the jury is likely to give too much credence to the apparent scientific validity of the numbers when, in fact, much judgment is required for their proper interpretation, (2) many persons, especially many lawyers, are not able to deal with or present statistical evidence competently and to put it into proper perspective, and (3) a statistical association *per se* tells us nothing about the actual relationship between the two events under consideration, and the law is more comfortable with "at least the illusion" of specific evidence linking the two, even though it comes through testimony that is no more credible than the statistical association. While Harter's statements reveal some of his own ignorance of the methodology and interpretation of statistical reasoning, there is much truth in what he says. Statistical data point to the probability of a cause-and-effect relationship but don't prove it. However, if that probability falls far beyond the role of a chance association and the evidence has a sound biological basis, there is good reason to give it careful consideration. This is particularly so if it conforms to the criteria for causation on epidemiological grounds to be discussed later in this chapter. These differing viewpoints as to what constitutes causal evidence in medicine and in law may result in quite different answers as to what is the cause of a disease or injury. In law, causation requires a higher order of proof and involves factors in addition to those usually required in establishing causation in medicine. At times these considerations seem scientifically unsound or capricious. There certainly appear to be deficiencies in the process as currently practiced in toxic tort cases. These include the failure to provide guidelines or standards as to what constitutes a "preponderance of evidence" and for defining what requirements are needed to designate a person as an "expert." Too often, physicians with no epidemiological or statistical training or experience are selected as experts. While courts are now more often admitting epidemiological evidence, rarely is that evidence used as the primary determinant of the decision.

Guidelines for Causation in Occupational Diseases

In his Presidential Address before the Section of Occupational Medicine of the Royal Society of Medicine in England in 1965, Sir Bradford Hill suggested a set of "viewpoints" as to whether the association between some aspect of the environment and a disease represented merely an association or a causal relationship. These are listed in Table 10.3 and are similar to the guidelines of the USPHS Surgeon-General's Report on Smoking and Lung Cancer published in January 1964 (Surgeon General, 1964). *Strength of the association* heads both lists and is reflected by the difference in rates between those exposed to an environmental or occupational toxin and those not exposed. However, it is seldom fulfilled for diseases like occupational cancer and for this reason was omitted from Doll's later criteria (Doll, 1985). Rare cancers like cancer of the scrotum or nasal sinuses or angiosarcoma of the liver may be increased in risk in

Table 10.3
Nine Viewpoints as to Whether Association
Means Causation[a]

Strength of the association
Consistency of association
Specificity of association
Temporality
Biological gradient
Plausibility
Coherence
Experiment
Analogy

[a]From Hill (1965).

appropriately exposed populations hundreds of times over that of the general population without affecting more than 1% of the work force, but the occurrence of even three or four cases in a few hundred employees constitutes such strong evidence that it effectively rules out any explanation other than that of cause and effect. In addition to the rarity of disease, as it contributes to the strength of the association, is the uniqueness of the exposure. For example, the surgeon Percival Pott in 1775 found an enormous increase in the risk of scrotal cancer among chimney sweeps. This risk persisted to as late as the second decade of the 20th century when the mortality from this cancer was still 200 times that of workers not so exposed to tar or mineral oils (Doll, 1964). Other examples of a high risk of disease in exposed versus nonexposed person, which is accompanied by a relatively low risk of disease within the exposed group, is the occurrence of lung cancer in smokers: here the risk is increased 32 times in doctors who smoke 25 cigarettes or more daily as compared with the nonsmoker, yet the actual incidence of lung cancer is only 2.27 per 1000 for heavy smokers as compared with 0.07 for the nonsmoking physician. The occurrence of a low incidence of clinical disease following an appropriate exposure to the causal agent is, of course, a well-known phenomenon in infectious diseases, like poliomyelitis and viral hepatitis, where only a very small percentage of those infected will become clinically ill. In the classical study of Snow (1855) on the transmission of cholera by water, he found a 14-fold difference in the cholera mortality rate in households supplied by water from a polluted part of the Thames River as compared with that for water obtained above the source of contamination, yet the actual death rates per 10,000 were only 71 and 5, respectively. Proper case–control studies of this type that show differences (relative risks or odds ratios) of 2 or greater are suggestive of a real risk and those over 10 are generally strong enough to compensate for errors in design. These include the exclusion of chance, of confounding, and consideration of the intensity, duration, and time of exposure. However, as in all case–control studies, the selection of the appropriate control group is both important and critical to the conclusions drawn. Gross differences in rates of incidence of a disease in a specific occupational group may be seen depending on whether the comparison group is selected on a national basis, a regional or local basis, or actual comparison with nonexposed persons in the same environment. While the greater selectivity and specificity in better-matched controls gives more meaningful comparisons, it also reduces the number of persons available for control so that valid statistical calculations may not be possible. The time–dosage relationship is very important in estimating causality as is the dose–response curve. These criteria may not always reflect the actual risk or be consistent for the duration of exposure, however. Doll has pointed out that the highest risk may be encountered for the shortest term worker for reasons that are not entirely clear, although the selection of appropriately matched controls may be one factor. In general, the relative risk between the exposed and the nonexposed worker or the general population is of much more importance in legal causation than the absolute differences in rates between them.

Consistency, the next on the list of Hill's viewpoints, refers to the need for similar findings by different investigators and by different techniques. Impressive in demonstrating this consistency was the relationship between smoking and lung cancer found in 29 retrospective and 7 prospective investigations completed at the time of Hill's 1965 paper. Since then, there have been many more confirmatory studies with the same results. However, there are situations in which repetition may not be possible because of the uniqueness of the exposure. The atomic exposure at Hiroshima is an example of this. Another would be a situation in which a change in the occupation or the environment removed the risk factor. Hill (1965) quotes a study of workers in nickel refineries in South Wales in which 16 of 1000 workers developed cancer of the lung and 11 developed cancer of the nasal sinuses (the death rates for all other cancers were similar.). The exposed group was limited to those working with chemical processes. After certain changes were made in the refining process, no further cases developed in persons employed after that time. Thus, repetition of the study was impossible. More than twenty years have passed since Hill's paper.

Specificity was the next viewpoint in which the association with the presumed exposure should be limited to specific workers and to particular sites and types of disease and without association with other causes of morbidity and mortality. At the same time, Hill recognized that diseases may have more than one cause. *Temporality* was his fourth viewpoint and indicated that the horse should precede the cart, i.e., the presumed exposure or cause in that particular occupation should precede the onset of the disease in that particular individual. This may not be so easy to establish if exposures occur both within and without the industry, or there are multiple causes of the same clinical disease, or in which the objective evidence of exposure and of the time–dosage relationship may have occurred years before. These relationships and their magnitude may be difficult to establish in the usual case–control, retrospective study. The *biological gradient* came next, and in Hill's view, reflected the need for a dose–response relationship, whereas *plausibility* dealt with the biological basis for the relationship between cause and effect. Others use the term "biological gradient" more to describe the array of severity of symptoms, ranging from none to death, that may follow exposure to an agent, and which in infectious diseases, as well as some chronic diseases, depend on the characteristics and the susceptibility of the host, as much as on the dosage and duration of the exposure. The biological basis for cause and effect is important to understand but sometimes this knowledge comes only after a strong enough association has been demonstrated to stimulate studies of possible pathogenesis. On the other hand, Hill emphasized under the criteria *coherence* that even a strong association should be viewed with suspicion if it seriously conflicts with the recognized natural history and biology of the disease. Laboratory studies may add to the coherence of the causal relationship, but the lack of data such as the inability to reproduce a disease in an animal should not eliminate the possibility that a real causal relationship exists: this same exception was made by Koch in his original postulates, as cholera, leprosy, and diphtheria, whose causative agents fulfilled the first two postulates, could not be reproduced in an experimental animal. Under his eighth viewpoint, Hill used *experiment* to indicate that the removal of the suspected cause should lower the frequency of the disease. Many of us would regard "experiment" as more properly applied to the experimental reproduction of the disease in an experimental animal. Finally, he said that *analogy* might lead to causal inferences. For example, the discovery that use of the tranquilizer thalidomide in pregnancy and that rubella infection during early pregnancy led to congenital abnormalities, might lead one to suspect that other drugs or other infections might behave similarly. While Hill suggested that his nine viewpoints (or criteria) of association deserved investigation before deciding on causation, he cautioned that he did not believe that any hard-and-fast rules of evidence *must* be obeyed before accepting a cause-and-effect relationship. Indeed, he went on to the further disclaimer that none of the nine viewpoints could bring reputable evidence for or against a causal hypothesis and none can be required as a *sine qua non*. In the more than 25 years since Hill's paper, the essential validity and usefulness of the viewpoints have, in my opinion, been reaffirmed as general guidelines for causation, as have those of the Surgeon General's criteria included in the 1964 report on smoking (Surgeon General, 1964). I feel that Hill was both too modest and too self-effacing about his "Viewpoints." Hill was a great biostatistician, yet declared that formal tests of significance cannot answer these questions of cause and effect, but can and should remind us of the role that chance can play and the magnitude of such effects. Indeed, he goes further to say that there are many situations in which the weight of epidemiological evidence is great enough or little enough that tests of significance are totally unnecessary. Two of his quotes on this issue of excessive emphasis on statistics are memorable: "What is worse, the glitter of the t table diverts attention from the inadequacy of the fare" and "Like fire, the χ^2 test is an excellent servant and bad master." I have devoted much time on Hill's paper because it, and the report of the Surgeon General (1964), represented brilliant codifications of the concepts of causation. They were important contributions to approaching the problem of causality in occupational exposures, or indeed in any cause-and-effect relationship.

Twenty years after Hill's important paper in 1965, another outstanding English epidemiologist, Sir Richard Doll, suggested another set of criteria for establishing a causal relationship in occupation (Doll, 1985). In this case, the causal exposure was to a presumed carcinogen and the effect was a malignant disease. They are listed in Table 10.4 and some of their epidemiological implications have already been discussed in this chapter. It deserves renotice that *strength of association* was omitted from the list simply because Doll felt that it was too seldom observed to be featured among the criteria. Included on his list was the need for *proper methodology* and for a demonstrable *dose–duration response,* and the requirement for consistency of the results obtained under different circumstances. However, he did not mention, as Hill had, the viewpoints of biological plausibility, coherence with the natural history of the disease, the induction of the disease in an experimental animal, or that removal of the suspected cause should lower the incidence of the disease. However, Doll's paper was more directed at the problems and biases inherent in epidemiological studies and at the proper interpretation of the evidence, than it was with setting forth a specific set of guidelines.

Table 10.4
Requirements for Establishing Carcinogenicity from Epidemiological Evidence According to Doll[a]

Positive association between exposure and disease in groups of individuals with known exposure (case–control or cohort studies) that:

(1) Is not explicable by bias in recording or detection, confounding, or chance.
(2) Varies appropriately with intensity and duration of exposure after exposure begins and ends.
(3) Is observed repeatedly in different circumstances.

[a]From Doll (1985).

In his paper on "The Dilemma of Causation in Toxic Torts," Harter (1985, 1986) indicates that once an association between an event and an injury or illness has been established, certain criteria be used to guide the judgment as to whether the events are causally related. The criteria he suggests are similar to those included in Hill's (1965) viewpoints and in the Surgeon General's (1964) report, such as strength of association, consistency of association, correct timing, specificity of association, biological gradient, biological plausibility, and prevalence and exposure. He states "These criteria are used to determine whether members of an exposed group are more likely to develop the disease than those who were not." According to him, causality is then expressed as the probability of incurring the disease following exposure. He points out that only rarely can it be scientifically determined who has had a particular disease because of exposure to a particular agent.

Bert Black, a lawyer, and David Lilienfeld, an epidemiologist, have proposed another set of guidelines that need to be fulfilled for epidemiological proof in toxic tort litigation (Black and Lilienfeld, 1984). They term the guidelines the "Henle–Koch–Evans" postulates. They represent what I termed, with tongue-in-cheek, a "Unified Concept of Causation" (Evans, 1976). There are reproduced with some modification by them in Table 10.5. They have been discussed in Chapter 5 and embody, in different terms, many of the thoughts included in Hill's (1965) paper, although I was not aware of his publication at the time I wrote mine. Black and Lilienfeld (1984) rightly point out that the postulates do not, by themselves, provide a complete legal standard because causation in law requires consideration of the degree of certainty required to meet the plaintiff's burden of proof. They suggest that this deficiency can be remedied by requiring that, in addition to the postulates, the concept of attributable risk be added: this should be greater than 50% for the factor in question. In this way, they would meet the legal requirement of "more likely than not." They state "If, in an exposed population, more than half the cases of a disease can be attributed to the exposure, and if the postulates are satisfied, then absent other information about a diseased individual, it is more likely than not his or her illness was caused by that exposure." It should be emphasized that stating that more than half the cases should be due to the exposure is not the same as saying that more than 50% of those exposed developed the disease. The latter rarely occurs in chronic or malignant disease, and is limited to highly toxic exposures resulting in a disease with a short incubation period, such as the cyanide exposure in the recent Bhopal incident in India. While I endorse these considerations in general, I feel that the postulates should be used primarily as a guide in seeking the "cause in fact" and the "preponderance of evidence" that the agent was "more likely than not" the cause of the disease; these constitute the legal requirements for establishing the causal proof. The failure to fulfill one or more of the postulates should not eliminate the possibility that such a relationship exists.

Table 10.5
The Henle–Koch–Evans Postulates[a]

1. The prevalence of the disease should be significantly higher in those exposed to the hypothesized cause than in controls not so exposed (the cause may be present in the external environment or as a defect in host responses).

2. Exposure to the hypothesized cause should be more frequent among those with the disease than in controls without the disease when all other risk factors are held constant.

3. Incidence of the disease should be significantly higher in those exposed to the cause than in those not so exposed, as shown by prospective studies.

4. Temporally, the disease should follow exposure to the hypothesized causative agent with the distribution of incubation periods as a log-normal-shaped curve.

5. A spectrum of host responses should follow exposure to the hypothesized agent along a logical biological gradient from mild to severe.

6. A measurable host response following exposure to the hypothesized cause should have a high probability of appearing in those lacking this response before exposure (e.g., antibody, cancer cells) or should increase in magnitude if present before exposure; this response pattern should occur infrequently in persons not so exposed.

7. Experimental reproduction of the disease should occur more frequently in animals or man appropriately exposed to the hypothesized cause than in those not so exposed; this exposure may be deliberate in volunteers, experimentally induced in the laboratory, or demonstrated in a controlled regulation of natural exposure.

8. Elimination or modification of the hypothesized cause or of the vector carrying it should decrease the incidence of the disease (e.g., control of polluted water, removal of tar from cigarettes).

9. Prevention or modification of the host's response on exposure to the hypothesized cause should decrease or eliminate the disease (e.g., immunization, drugs to lower cholesterol, specific lymphocyte transfer factor in cancer).

10. All of the relationships and findings should make biological and epidemiological sense.

[a]From Black and Lilienfeld (1984).

In a paper presented at a conference on "Causation and Financial Compensation" held in 1984, I presented a modification of my "Unified Concept of Causation" as adapted to occupational exposures (Evans, 1986). These are listed in Table 10.6 in a slightly modified form. They combine features of several of the viewpoints and guidelines already discussed. The first five are designed to determine if the risk of developing the disease is greater in those exposed in an occupational setting as compared with those not so exposed and to show that this risk increases with the intensity and duration of the exposure. Such differences should be statistically significant and the relative risk should be at least 2 or more to suggest causality. The proof would involve retrospective and prospective studies in several settings and by several investigators to render them meaningful. Both the absolute and the relative risk of exposure should be measured, if possible, and the risk attributable to that particular exposure calculated. The

Table 10.6
Postulates of Causation for Occupational Disease[a]

1. *Prevalence* of the disease should be higher in those exposed to the putative causes in an occupational setting than in those not so exposed either in the same setting or other similar settings; if possible, this should be shown in matched controls.
2. *Exposure* to the putative cause should be clearly demonstrated by historical and/or laboratory data to have occurred more often in those with the disease than in those without the disease when all other factors are held constant and be shown more likely than not to have caused the disease.
3. *Risk* of developing the disease should increase with the duration and intensity of exposure to the putative cause.
4. *Incidence* of the disease should be higher in those exposed to the putative cause than in those not so exposed as shown in prospective studies.
5. *Temporally* the disease should follow exposure to the putative cause in that workplace and both exposure and disease should be absent prior to starting work in that workplace.
6. *Other causes* of the same disease outside the workplace should be excluded or, if present, the attributable risk of each exposure assessed.
7. A *biological gradient* of response to the putative cause should regularly appear or should increase following exposure to the putative causes as shown by objective evidence.
8. *Elimination or modification* of the putative cause, or the vehicle carrying it, or protection of the worker against it, should decrease the incidence of the disease.
9. *Experimental reproduction* of the disease should be demonstrated, if possible, in susceptible animals or humans exposed accidentally or deliberately to the putative cause.
10. *The relationship* between cause and effect should be shown in several studies, make biological and epidemiological sense, and be consistent with the natural history of the disease.

[a]From Evans, 1986 (with permission).

contribution, if any, of exposure to the same or other causes of the same disease outside the workplace should be examined. The cause should be shown to precede the effect, and a biological gradient of response should be demonstrated. The removal, modification, or control of the exposure should decrease the frequency of the disease. Exposure of animals to the presumed cause should result in the same disease, or this should be shown in "experiments in nature" in which some individuals are exposed and other comparable persons are not. The relationship between cause and effect should make, or later be shown to make, biological and epidemiological sense and be consistent with the natural history of the disease. These postulates or guidelines, as true of the others presented, were not, and are not intended to be, rigid criteria for causation but simply a framework in which the "cause in fact" can be pursued.

Limitations and Applications

Epidemiology is often defined as the study of the determinants of health and disease in population groups (MacMahon *et al.*, 1960) reflecting the Greek *epi* ("on") and *demos* ("the people"). The sequence of evidence in toxic tort cases as outlined in Table 10.7 first involves the proof of "cause in fact." The evidence to support this is that exposure to cause A led to disease B in individual C. This need for specificity of each element is not reflected by the general guidelines of epidemiological causation in which the risk (or probability) of developing disease B following exposure to cause A is significantly higher (risk 2× or more) in *groups* of exposed persons than that found in controls, ideally represented by nonexposed matched controls but often by the risk in the general population. They are also interested in the degree to which that cause resulted in that disease in groups of persons (the attributable risk) when other causes of the same disease are excluded. Cigarette smoking, for example, accounts for about 70% of the cases of lung cancer and other causes for the rest. The emphasis in these considerations is on groups of persons. Legal requirements are concerned with the risk in the *individual*, the plaintiff, and whether the preponderance of evidence supports the conclusion that *that* exposure "more likely than not" resulted in *that* illness or injury in *that* person. This is a much higher order of proof and specificity than involved in most epidemiological proof and classically it must be shown that the disease would not have occurred "but for" the particular exposure. This criterion was later modified to the exposure being "a substantial" factor bringing about the disease or injury. Neither epidemiological nor legal proof often considers the role of individual susceptibility in their criteria of proof, probably because it is so difficult to measure. But it is clear that only some persons exposed to exactly the same cause in the same dosage will develop the disease while the

Table 10.7
Summary of the Legal Chain of Causation and Compensation

1. Plaintiff claims that exposure to cause A in the workplace produced disease B.
2. "Cause in fact" must be shown by a preponderance of evidence that cause A more likely than not produced disease B (preferably that it was a necessary and sufficient cause).
3. If other causes of disease B exist to which the plaintiff was also exposed either prior to entry or outside the workplace, then the risk attributable to each must be determined.
4. The plaintiff must show that the action of the defendant was a substantial factor in bringing about the result.
5. "Proximate cause," a legal and policy determination, must be judged and involves the liability of the defendant; it is usually based on the demonstration that the "cause in fact" increased the risk of the disease or injury and that this risk was a reasonably foreseeable one.
6. The amount of financial compensation must be determined by the court based ideally on the attributable risk of the disease due to cause A, the degree of liability of the defendant for permitting a foreseeable risk, and the medical costs involved. Often costs for "pain and suffering" and "punitive costs" are included in this judgment.

majority will not. I have called such influences "the clinical illness promotion factor(s)" (Evans, 1985) and they are discussed in the next chapter. Their existence complicates both the judgment of legal issues of "cause in fact" and "proximate cause" in terms of liability for the exposure, as well as whether the risk was a reasonably foreseeable one. AIDS is a good example of the effect of altered susceptibility on the occurrence of diseases that are usually due to organisms that are not pathogenic in normal persons. These limitations in the availability or application of epidemiological and other scientific evidence in establishing causation in the individual in toxic law cases have resulted in limited usage in courts and in questions of their ability to meet the legal requirements of proof. Thus, these shortcomings have sometimes led to evidence other than scientific in legal decisions. As Harter (1985) has stated: "The decisions in toxic tort cases, therefore, are based on policy as well as science, at least in the face of scientific uncertainty." The issue of judging causation in law is clearly compounded by the need for expert epidemiological judgment by persons untrained in that science— the jury, judge, and often the lawyers. The "expert witnesses" often fulfill no standard requirements of training and/or experience and because they are hired by the plaintiff or the defendant they are apt to present the evidence favorable to their client. In this way, whatever truth may exist may be pushed out of context by adversarial presentations. One lawyer recently went so far as to state that the tort system is not really concerned with causation but is a form of guerilla warfare (Marshaw, 1986). In addition to causation, the court must judge the presence and magnitude of liability involved, the extent of injury or disease in the plaintiff, the cost of medical care necessary to treat it (including "pain and punishment"), and the financial compensation to be awarded. These are formidable challenges and the modifications of the system needed to improve it may be very difficult to carry out.

Current Examples of Toxic Tort Litigation

Some examples of current toxic tort cases are given in Table 10.8. They have arisen from exposures in the environment, in occupations, in pharmaceutical plants, and in various consumer-related issues. The proof of causation in some of the cases is meager, falling short of both the epidemiological and the legal criteria. Included in this are exposures involving a large number of persons, several types of presumed disease consequences, large financial claims, eager lawyers, often working on contingency fees, and court costs so high that in some instances it is deemed cheaper to set up a compensation fund for all those exposed who developed some subsequent illness, than to settle the cases individually. Examples of this are Love Canal, the Three Mile Island nuclear power plant, and Agent Orange. The interest in these exposures and their possible disease consequences have been greatly exaggerated by the press, leading to extensive litigation and class action suits. On the other hand, there are suits in which the causal evidence seems very strong, such as exposures to asbestos, cyanide, and vinyl chloride in occupational settings, consumer claims for injuries or disease from use of the Dalkon shield, certain types of tampons in relation to the toxic shock syndrome, and the reactions to various vaccines such as swine influenza, pertussis, and oral poliomyelitis. In some of these examples, the risk

Table 10.8
Examples of Recent Toxic Tort Cases

Environmental/occupational	Consumer-related
Agent Orange	Dalkon shield
Digoxin	Influenza swine flu vaccine
Love Canal	Pertussis vaccine
Three Mile Island nuclear power plant	Toxic shock syndrome

was foreseeable, as in the case of asbestos and cyanide, but in others it did not appear until the product was actually in use, such as the swine flu vaccine, the Rely brand of Tampon, and congenital defects from ingestion of thalidomide taken during pregnancy. In other instances, the risk is foreseeable, albeit often miniscule, but is unavoidable because it is an inherent property of the preparation itself, and not due to negligence on the part of the manufacturer. These include vaccines like oral poliomyelitis and pertussis, and many pharmaceutical preparations. The dispensing physician is often sued in these cases for failing to warn the patient adequately about the possible side effects of the preparation. This places an enormous burden on the physician since almost all vaccines and drugs can result in side reactions or complications, and to list all possible ones would entail so much of the physician's time that little would be left for other patients. For example, in the United States, the incidence of paralytic poliomyelitis following the oral vaccine is estimated as 1 per 11.5 million recipients and 1 per 1 million contacts of vaccinated persons (Melnick, 1989). Should the physician spend the time to discuss this remote risk with the 3 to 11 million patients who are to receive oral vaccine, when only one may develop the complication, and when the risk of having an automobile accident en route to the physician may be of a higher magnitude? The use of a printed informed consent form may help save the physician's time under some circumstances. The risks of litigation for the physician and the manufacturer associated with vaccines probably require backup with government insurance or production of the vaccine itself by a government agency, if the interests in protecting the public against preventable infectious diseases are to succeed. The issue now becomes even more complicated because most states require evidence of immunization against certain specified diseases including DPT, measles, and poliomyelitis as a condition to entry into the primary school system, and many colleges are now requiring proof of measles immunization before starting school. There is obviously a legal conflict between mandatory immunization and the liability of the rare consequences of the procedure itself. The same issue of informed consent exists in the Armed Forces where certain immunizations are required on entry into the service and periodically thereafter, and may include unusual vaccinations, as well as prophylactic drugs to protect the soldier in tropical areas.

Space does not permit discussion of the causal evidence for or against most of these large-scale toxic tort cases, or class action suits, but two examples are briefly summarized below.

Agent Orange

The use of the defoliant Agent Orange, which contains dioxin, during the Vietnam conflict by U.S. armed forces personnel has led to many epidemiological studies of the possible toxic effects of such exposure, and many legal claims have been made based on a wide variety of diseases that presumably were due to this exposure. Such studies include a comparison of all diseases subsequently appearing in airplane crews who were heavily exposed during dissemination of the agent with crews of cargo planes in the same environment not so exposed. The result of this investigation showed no significant difference between the two groups in the incidence of any chronic or malignant disease with the possible exception of chloracne, a disease of the skin that is not disabling or fatal. The distinguished judge Jack B. Weinstein of the U.S. District Court for the Eastern District of New York has brilliantly reviewed all of the data and concluded that there is no evidence of a causal association (Weinstein, 1984). Yet despite the lack of epidemiological proof, the government has set up a $180 million settlement fund to pay for all claims that fulfill the following criteria: (1) proven exposure, (2) claim does not involve traumatic or accidental injury, (3) age not over 60, (4) payment only for death or total disability. This action would seem to fly in the face of scientific and epidemiological evidence. This may create an unfortunate precedent in which compensation is paid without examining causality. In a more recent evaluation of the feasibility of epidemiological studies of Agent Orange, the Centers for Disease Control, on orders from Congress, examined the problem in persons in III Corp's tactical zone, an area of the heaviest spraying of the defoliant (Booth, 1988). They found that levels of dioxin in the blood of "exposed" veterans in this area between 1967 and 1968 were low, and similar to unexposed controls serving stateside and in Germany. They also found it impossible to measure the degree of individual exposure accurately because of poor records on distribution of Agent Orange, and because spraying was irregular and ubiquitous, and the military records of the soldiers themselves were inadequate to the task of identifying illness. Thus, problems both of dosage of the agent and of the degree of host response confounded the study, and CDC felt such a study to be both difficult and expensive, if not impossible.

Swine Flu Vaccine and the Guillain–Barre Syndrome

Influenza is one of the great, unconquered epidemic diseases, now second only to the epidemic of AIDS, in terms of world impact. Despite WHO's establishment of laboratories around the world, so-called "listening posts," that are able to recognize new strains and early epidemics of the virus, worldwide epidemics still occur because it takes at least 6 months to prepare even a few million doses of vaccine from the new strains. One of the most devastating of the influenza epidemics, or of any epidemic disease in history, was the influenza outbreak beginning in 1918, in which half the world was infected and 20 million people died. It is no wonder, then, that the isolation of a virus that resembled the 1918 strain in a small group of recruits at Fort Dix, New Jersey caused great concern among public health personnel. Its resemblance to the great epidemic strain was based on antibody studies alone since the first influenza virus ever isolated was the swine strain in 1931 by Shope. While this strain was derived from an Iowa pig and the original virus may have persisted in this species ever since, there had been a few human cases from contact with infected pigs, but no human epidemic from this strain in the intervening years between the pandemic and the Fort Dix episode. Did the occurrence in a small epidemic in humans presage the development of a new pandemic or was it the result of some special feature of the recruit population in whom close contact may have fostered the spread of a virus that was of low epidemicity? This was the question faced by the experts. If the answer was yes, then the New Jersey virus was already on hand to make vaccine quickly and possibly prevent a major epidemic. Five experts estimated the probability as 0.10 (range 0.02 to 0.25); if the epidemic were to occur, it would cause an estimated 60 million cases of swine influenza and 50,000 excess deaths (Langmuir et al., 1984). On this basis a mass immunization program was recommended to President Ford, who approved it, and Congress authorized $135 million for its execution, which began on October 1, 1976. No epidemic occurred and the vaccine was followed by cases of Guillain–Barre syndrome (GBS), a usually benign disease of the central nervous system but sometimes producing permanent paralysis or even death. This has led to much criticism of the decision, its method of implementation, and to many court suits against the government who provided reinsurance to the manufacturers. The complications received great publicity in the press and other media. The mass vaccination program was discontinued in mid-December, 1976, after 45 million doses had been given. While I personally believe the decision was the correct one under the circumstances and that the expenditure of $135 million represented an insurance-type policy against a catastrophic event that did not occur (Evans, 1977), I cannot argue with critics on the poor way some aspects of the vaccine's administration were handled, especially the lack of an adequate surveillance system to report diseases that followed vaccination as compared with an unvaccinated group. However, the risk of GBS was not really a foreseeable one, as it had never been a major complication of influenza vaccines (although it did occur rarely after many types of immunization, as well as after many infectious diseases), and no such intense and mass vaccination of influenza had ever been carried out before. The causal association between the vaccine and GBS became a matter of intensive epidemiological investigation and of legal action. Through 1984, over 4000 claims totaling over $3 billion pertaining to a variety of conditions presumably resulting from the vaccine had been submitted (Langmuir et al., 1984). An increased risk of GBS in the 8 to 10 weeks following vaccination had been found as compared with nonvaccinated groups (Langmuir, 1984;

Schonberger *et al.*, 1979) but criticisms of the studies led U.S. District Court Judge Gerhard in November 1981 to order the release of the data underlying these reports to the plaintiffs in the cases. This prompted the creation of a special scientific panel to reevaluate the data released. Their report, published in 1984 (Langmuir *et al.*, 1984), indicated that the more severe cases of GBS suggested a causal relationship between the disease and the vaccine whereas cases with limited motor involvement showed no such pattern. The increased risk in the more severe cases lasted for at least 6 weeks after vaccination, possibly 8 weeks, but no longer. The relative risk in the 6-week period of vaccinated versus unvaccinated persons ranged from 3.96 to 7.75 depending on the baseline estimate of incidence in the unvaccinated. Under their estimate, from 211 to 246 cases of GBS were attributable to the vaccine above the normal risk. The total rate of GBS among vaccinees ranged from 4.9 to 5.9 per million persons vaccinated. The risk was thus not far from that mentioned for paralysis after oral polio vaccine. The unusual causal aspects of the association between swine flu vaccine and GBS are that the Henle–Koch postulates were not fulfilled, the actual "cause" involved—some unknown ingredient contained in the vaccine—was not identified, the causal relationship was limited to a period of not greater than 8 weeks, appeared to exist only for the more severe form of the syndrome, and has not followed the administration of other influenza vaccines subsequent to the discontinuance of swine flu vaccine in recipients kept under close surveillance for the possible occurrence of such complications. In addition, the biological basis for causation has not been established, although some type of immunological sensitization of T lymphocytes to a component of the vaccine that results in injury to nerve tissue seems a good possibility. The swine flu episode reflects the very specialized nature of the circumstances of the exposure and of the disease that presumably resulted from swine flu vaccine and the complexities in trying to establish a scientific basis for causation. To make matters even worse, one of the members of the expert panel who signed the report now doubts the validity of the conclusions because he can find no evidence that GBS followed swine flu vaccination in members of the armed forces who were vaccinated at the same time as the civilian population and in whom the recognition of at least more severe cases of GBS should be high (Kurland *et al.*, 1985).

Possible Modifications of the System

The goals of the tort system, according to Harter (1985, 1986), are to reduce the aggregate social cost of illnesses resulting from toxic materials, both in preventing the disease and in compensating persons in whom it has occurred. The costs must be fair and equitable. The evidence of causation required by the legal system in individual cases is of such a high order and the circumstances under which the judgment must be made so adverse that it is very difficult, if not impossible, to achieve the goals set forth by Harter. What can be done to modify the system or to find an alternative system as used in other countries?

Within the current system one might require two things: (1) the use of a set of standard guidelines in assembling evidence for "cause in fact" and for determination of "attributable risk", (2) the assignment of judgment of cause in fact to an independent group of well-established experts. The former might involve a set of standards agreed upon by a panel from the American Bar Association and the American College of Epidemiology. As most of the guidelines presented in this chapter are based on very similar principles, it should not be an impossible task. Available lists on the known occupational toxins that can produce chronic or malignant diseases and the degree and time of exposure estimated as necessary to produce the effect should be assembled and used in determining attributable risk. The use of established postulates of causation and of measuring attributable risk has been recommended by Black and Lilienfeld (1984). The use of an expert, administrative panel to judge the evidence for causality and compensation based on attributable risk has been suggested by Elliot (1986), who also recommends that punitive damages be prohibited. Harter (1985, 1986) has also endorsed the concept of a panel of experts to "review the scientific claims of causality and to weed out the patently frivolous" but feels that the maintenance of a high-quality panel would not only be expensive but would not address the societal issue of whom to compensate. In my view, the cost issue must be judged in relation to the high cost of the current system, in which some 60% of the total expenditures are administrative and much money goes to legal fees. As to Harter's second reservation, I feel that the issue of liability compensation should be left to the court, which will hopefully eliminate the punitive and pain and suffering costs. Greater use of negotiation rather than litigation would also be useful, as suggested by Eads (1986), and one might hope that the motivation and reward for "contingency" fees paid to lawyers will be reduced. One alternative suggested by Marshaw (1986) is a compensation fund in which risks are pooled without worrying about the issue of causation per se—a socialized risk system related to the disability encountered. Some system like the current "no-fault" automobile insurance compensation might be tried.

Legal systems other than our own deserve examination for possible solutions to our current dilemma. As discussed by Prichard (1986), dean of the Toronto Law School, England's system differs from ours in four respects: (1) the greater economic incentives in toxic tort cases in the U.S., (2) the greater use of class action suits in the U.S., (3) the higher payments for compensation in the U.S., (4) the lower number of criteria for legal causation employed here. In New Zealand, compensation is paid without regard to cause in cases of injury resulting from automobile and occupational accidents but does not apply to diseases, which are handled by a quasi-governmental body. Claims are made by an insurance mechanism until the need for submission to court becomes necessary. Payment schedules are set up to pay for 100% of reasonable medical costs and a certain amount of liability. The funding for this compensation varies: to help pay for injuries caused by automobiles, a levy (currently about $21.00) is made on car owners; for occupational accidents the employers of the injured worker(s) pay a small amount each payroll period, similar to our workmen's compensation; for other groups payment is made out of general taxation funds with no levy on the manufacturer.

These suggestions do not reflect the more conservative recommendations of the panel members who wrote the final report for the "Conference on Causation and Financial Compensation" (Novey, 1986), which are given below in abbreviated form:

1. Society should seek to articulate clearer legal concepts and guidelines regarding what must be demonstrated about causation to justify an award of compensation or to impose responsibility for funding compensation.
2. The scientific community should seek ways to develop and explain scientific information so as to provide the most useful assistance to the legal system in making compensation and funding decisions.
3. Judges should endeavor to learn more about the nature of scientific controversy and what is within the realm of sound scientific methodology and reasoning. They should take a more active role to exclude expert opinion based on unsound scientific methodology and reasoning and to scrutinize who is or is not an expert in the field—yet without depriving the jury of its essential task of deciding cases where there is a genuine difference of sound scientific opinion.
4. Major improvements will likely come not so much from trying to change the application of causation requirements under the tort system as from more fundamental and structural reform of present compensation and litigation processes.
5. One potentially important group of possible improvements would not address causation directly but would change the incentives and environment of litigation to improve the functioning of the tort system overall.
6. Another kind of possible improvement would be the establishment of alternatives to the traditional tort remedy. Such alternative remedies should be developed at least for mass-disaster tort situations and should be considered for broader classes of toxic tort situations as well.
7. It is appropriate in an alternative compensation program to apply a relatively unrestricted concept of causation for determining eligibility, if causation is to be an eligibility criterion at all. However, general

"presumptions" of causation would establish a concept of causation that is too vague and inclusive for use in establishing eligibility to receive compensation from defendant companies.

8. Panels of medical and scientific experts might be effectively used to resolve causation issues under alternative compensation programs. Convening a panel of scientific experts cannot substitute for articulating a clear legal concept of causation, however. The experts' role would be to develop a rigorous scientific assessment, so that this assessment could be compared to the legal standard to see whether compensation should be paid.

9. It may be desirable to limit the traditional tort remedy to situations where both causation and fault are more clearly established than is now often required.

10. Increasing concern about the fairness and effectiveness of present arrangements for awarding compensation and assessing liability call for renewed consideration of a national health financing system or other national programs for protecting individuals against the financial impact of disease, disability, and death without regard to cause.

Summary

Our toxic tort system in the United States is regarded by many, including distinguished lawyers and judges, as impractical and outmoded. The legal standards of proof are too high, well-established guidelines to seek the "cause in fact" are not followed, attributable risk is often overlooked, the judgment of causation is made by juries untrained in such evaluation, evidence is presented in an adversarial manner by lawyers or by "experts" whose scientific and epidemiological expertise has not been adequately established, and contingency fees and financial issues often blur the scientific evidence. The awards for compensation often do not recognize pre-existing medical insurance or other plans that might reduce the award for medical care and may include high amounts for punitive damages and for pain and suffering. Several suggestions are made to modify the system, primarily the use of a set of standard guidelines of causation in seeking evidence for causation and of attributable risk and that independent groups of experts be employed to evaluate the evidence for "cause in fact," leaving the issues of liability and compensation to the court. Despite these views, some of which were also expressed by distinguished lawyers and judges in the 1985 conference on "Causation and Financial Compensation," the final conclusions and recommendations of the summarizing panel of four lawyers and one physician were more conservative than this, albeit making good suggestions for improvement in the tort system as currently practiced.

References

Armenian HK, Lilienfeld AM: The distribution of incubation periods of neoplastic diseases. *Am J Epidemiol* **99:**92–100, 1974.

Black B: Causation and case law—Where theory and practice diverge, in Novey LW (ed): *Causation and Financial Compensation*. Washington, DC, Georgetown University Medical Press, 1986, pp 233–242.

Black B, Lilienfeld DE: Epidemiological proof in toxic tort litigation. *Fordham Law Rev* **52:**723–785, 1984.

Booth W: Agent Orange hits back. *Science* **241:**1286–1288, 1988.

Brown C: Accident compensation in New Zealand, in Novey LW (ed): *Causation and Financial Compensation*. Washington, DC, Georgetown University Medical Press, 1986, pp 367–380.

Doll R: *Medical Surveys and Clinical Trials,* 2nd ed. Witts (ed). London, 1964, p 333.

Doll R: Occupational cancer: A hazard for epidemiologists. *Int J Cancer* **14:**22–31, 1985.

Eads GC: Designing safer products: Corporate responses to product liability law and regulation, in Novey LW (ed): *Causation and Financial Compensation*. Washington, DC, Georgetown University Medical Press, 1986, pp 335–344.

Elliot ED: What do we wish from the system? Of goals and institutional mismatches, in Novey LW (ed): *Causation and Financial Compensation*. Washington, DC, Georgetown University Medical Press, 1986, pp 268–288.

Evans AS: Causation and disease. The Henle–Koch postulates revisited. *Yale J Biol Med* **49:**175–195, 1976.

Evans AS: Editorial. Swine influenza program. *Yale J Biol Med* **50:**657–659, 1977.

Evans AS: The clinical illness promotion factor: A third ingredient. *Yale J Biol Med* **55:**193–199, 1985.

Evans AS: Causation in the biological sciences: Evolution of our concepts of causation and disease, in Novey LW (ed): *Causation and Financial Compensation*. Washington, DC, Georgetown University Medical Press, 1986, pp 155–174.

Gordis L: Causation in epidemiological studies, in Novey LW (ed): *Causation and Financial Compensation*. Washington, DC, Georgetown University Medical Press, 1986, pp 101–116.

Harter PJ: The dilemma of causation in toxic torts. Selected studies of health policy issues. Monograph 101. Washington, DC, Georgetown University Medical Press, 1985.

Harter PJ: The dilemma of causation in toxic torts, in Novey LW (ed): *Causation and Financial Compensation*. Washington, DC, Georgetown University Medical Press, 1986, pp 193–198.

Hill AB: The environment and disease: Association or causation? *Proc R Soc Med* **58:**295–300, 1965.

Kurland LT, Weiderholt WC, Kirpatrick JW, *et al:* Swine influenza vaccine and Guillain–Barre syndrome. Epidemic or artifact? *Arch Neurol* **42:**1089–1090, 1985.

Langmuir AD: Swine influenza virus incident (letter). *J R Soc Med* **77:**621, 1984.

Langmuir AD, Bregman DJ, Kurland LT, *et al:* An epidemiological and clinical analysis of Guillain–Barre syndrome reported in association with the administration of swine influenza vaccine. *Am J Epidemiol* **119:**841–879, 1984.

Lilienfeld AM, Lilienfeld DC: *The Foundations of Epidemiology,* 2nd ed. London, Oxford University Press, 1982.

MacMahon B, Pugh TFT, Ipsen J: *Epidemiologic Methods*. Boston, Little Brown & Co., 1960.

Marshaw J: A comment on causation reform and guerilla warfare, in Novey LW (ed): *Causation and Financial Compensation*. Washington, DC, Georgetown University Medical Press, 1986, pp 289–297.

Melnick J: Enteroviruses, in Evans AS (ed): *Viral Infections of Humans: Epidemiology and Control,* 3rd ed. New York, Plenum Press, 1989, pp 191–264.

Novey LB (ed): *Causation and Financial Compensation.* Washington, DC, Georgetown University Medical Press, 1986.

Prichard JRS: Why is American tort law so different? in Novey LW (ed): *Causation and Financial Compensation.* Washington, DC, Georgetown University Medical Press, 1986, pp 359–366.

Priest GL: Remarks of individual panel members, in Novey LW (ed): *Causation and Financial Compensation.* Washington, DC, Georgetown University Medical Press, 1986, pp 475–481.

Schonberger LB, Bregman DJ, Sullivan-Balyai JZ, *et al:* Guillain–Barre syndrome following vaccination in the national influenza immunization program, United States, 1976–77. *Am J Epidemiol* **110:**105–123, 1979.

Shope RE: Swine influenza. III. Filtration experiments with etiology. *J Exp Med* **54:**373–385, 1931.

Simonato G, Saracci R: Causes, occupational, in Parmeggiani L (ed): *Encyclopedia of Occupational Health and Safety.* Geneva, International Labor Office, Geneva, 1983.

Snow J: *On the Etiology of Cholera.* London, Commonwealth Press, 1855.

Surgeon General: Report of a committee on smoking and lung cancer. Washington, DC, USPHS, 1964.

Susser MW: Rules of inference in epidemiology, in Novey LW (ed): *Causation and Financial Compensation.* Washington, DC, Georgetown University Medical Press, 1986, pp 175–192.

Weil H: Asbestos associated diseases: Science and public policy. *Chest* **84:**601, 1983.

Weil H: Epidemiologic evidence of causation, in Novey LW (ed): *Causation and Financial Compensation.* Washington, DC, Georgetown University Medical Press, 1986, pp 133–138.

Weinstein J: Preliminary reflections on managing disasters. *Columbia J Environ Law* **1:**1–11, 1985.

Weinstein J: "Agent Orange" Product Liability, 611 F Suppl 1396 (ED, NY, 1984); In re "Agent Orange" Product Liability Litigation, 597 F Suppl 740 (ED, NY, 1984).

Weinstein J: The role of the court in toxic tort litigation, in Novey LW (ed): *Causation and Financial Compensation.* Washington, DC, Georgetown University Medical Press, 1986, pp 455–460.

11

The Clinical Illness Promotion Factor

A Third Ingredient

This monograph has focused largely on the establishment of the causal role of a given factor in the production of a disease or clinical syndrome by epidemiological and/or experimental means (Evans, 1976). This proof often included reproduction of the disease in a susceptible laboratory animal or susceptible human host (as per the Henle–Koch postulates), the demonstration that the disease occurs more commonly in the presence of the suspected factor than in its absence (increased relative risk), or that removal of the factor decreases the incidence of the disease (attributable risk). These approaches to causative proof have concentrated mainly on two ingredients: the suspected factor and the human host.

It is time we focus on clinical illness promotion factors as "a third ingredient." In his short story of that title, O. Henry (1937) relates the tale of a poor girl who has a piece of beef and a young man who has a potato. Together they join with these two ingredients to make a stew. It is clear, however, that a third ingredient is necessary to make a good stew. In this instance the essential third ingredient is an onion. The rest of the story concerns the search for someone with this ingredient. In epidemiological studies we should also be searching for a third ingredient. The admixture of a "causative agent" fully clothed with all of the potential antigens, oncogenic properties, or other putative pathogenetic factors necessary to produce disease with a fully susceptible host of the proper age, sex, socioeconomic, and nutritional status is often insufficient to result in clinical disease. A third ingredient, or even additional ones, may be needed. This is true

---

This chapter is reprinted from an article that appeared in the *Yale Journal of Biology and Medicine* (Evans AS: *Yale J Biol Med* **55**:193–199, 1982) by permission of the publisher.

Table 11.1
Third Ingredients: Factors That Might Influence the Occurrence and Severity
of Clinical Disease among Infected Persons

Age at the time of infection
Alcoholism
Anatomic defects
Antibiotic or antiviral resistance
Chronic disease: either pre- or coexisting
Dosage of organism
Double infections (viral, bacterial, parasitic, fungal)
Drugs: self- or physician-administered
Genetic makeup, especially effect on the immune system
Iatrogenic influences: other therapies, surgery, etc.
Immune status of host at time of infection
Immune response of host to infection (beneficial or detrimental)
Immunodeficiency: natural, drug-induced, disease-induced
Mechanism of disease production: lysis hypersensitivity, immune-complex
Mutation of organism during course of infection
Perception of illness by patient
Physical status at time of infection
Physical exercise during incubation period or at time of onset
Portal of entry of organism
Pregnancy
Psychosocial factors
Stress
Temperature of body at site of entry and viral multiplication
Trauma

---

of causative factors in both acute and chronic diseases. While the multifactorial origin of disease has been recognized by many authors, I wish to focus on the factor(s) that result in clinical disease among those exposed to all of the risk factors. This I will call "the third ingredient," or the clinical illness promotion factor (CIPF).

Acute Infectious Diseases

A major riddle in infectious diseases is why some individuals develop clinical illness as a result of infection while others do not. This variation in host response is true of most viral infections, although a few, such as rabies and measles infections, almost always result in clinical illness. Some of the clinical illness promotion factors influencing the host response are listed in Table 11.1. Age at the time of infection is one important determinant of the host response, especially to agents such as poliomyelitis virus, hepatitis A virus, and Epstein–Barr (EB) virus. With these agents, greater age of the host at the time of infection correlates with a greater possibility of clinical illness. Variations in the virulence of strains of virus, in the size of the inoculum, in the portal of entry, and in the status of the host have also been incriminated in producing clinical illness among those infected. Marked host variations exist, however, even when all of these factors are held constant. For example, hepatitis B virus contaminated one lot of yellow fever vaccine given to over 5000 healthy male soldiers of about the same age at Camp Polk. Each received the same dose in the same arm on the same day (Pan, 1945). Of those inoculated, 1004 (20%) developed clinical jaundice, and the rest did not. The incubation period from injection to clinical illness varied from 60 to 154 days (mean 96.4 days). What "third ingredient" influenced the variability in host response and incubation period among these soldiers? Unfortunately, we don't know the answer to this, since no studies were made to analyze this "natural experiment," and, even if they had been, the laboratory tools were not available at that time to identify susceptibility and immunity or to recognize subclinical infections.

A deliberate search for factors influencing EBV infection and disease [*clinical* infectious mononucleosis (IM)] was made among a single class of cadets at the West Point Military Academy studied over a four-year period (Hallee *et al.*, 1974; Kasl *et al.*, 1979). Psychosocial factors were measured on admission, and leadership and academic records were recorded during school. Among 432 susceptible cadets, 194 (44.9%) became infected over the four years, and 238 (55.1%) remained susceptible four years later (Hallee *et al.*, 1974). Among the 194 EBV-infected cadets, 48 developed clinical IM (24.7%) and 146 (75.3%) did not. The reasons for this difference were sought in psychosocial behavior patterns and in academic achievement. A high commitment to a military career was associated with a 57.1% clinical attack rate among EBV-infected cadets, and low military commitment with only a 10.7% rate of clinical IM. High military commitment influenced infection and disease in opposite directions, since it was associated with a *low infection* rate among susceptibles and *high clinical IM* rates among the infected. If one had not separately identified the susceptibles, the infected, and those with disease, this distinction would have been obscured. Academic performance also influenced the clinical attack rate in the third and fourth year. Those susceptible cadets whose academic performance was poorer in the second semester than in the first semester during the year prior to EBV seroconversion had a 50% clinical attack rate, as compared with only a 5.6% clinical attack rate in those with relatively good academic performance in the second semester compared with the first semester. The level of motivation toward a military career was inversely related to academic performance. Therefore, high motivation and poor academic performance correlated with high rates of clinical IM (43.5%). The serious, well-motivated student who failed in his academic expectations was, thus, especially susceptible to clinical illness after infection had occurred. This same student, however, was less apt to be exposed and infected. These studies indicate that if susceptibility, infection, and disease categories can be objectively identified, the clinical illness promotion factor—here, psychosocial factors—may emerge as a "third ingredient" rather than being obscured or diluted out by the presence of immune and unexposed individuals. It should be emphasized that the biological mechanisms by which psychosocial factors influence infection and disease in West Point cadets are not known, and these findings may not necessarily apply to other settings.

Genetics also play an important role in the response of the host to infection. Earlier investigations of twins and families had suggested that genetics played a role in the occurrence of paralysis in poliomyelitis (Reedy, 1957) and in the occurrence of rheumatic fever following Group A streptococcal infections (Wilson and Sweitzer, 1954). However, quantitative evaluation of exposure and the presence of prior immunity within family units were not adequately considered in these studies. More elegant were the twin and family analyses of Kallman and Reisner (1943) in tuberculosis, in which the corrected rates for *manifest* tuberculosis on exposure to an index case in the family were 7.1% in marriage partners, 11.9% in half-siblings, 25.5% in dizygotic co-twins, and 83.3% in monozygotic twins. More recently, the importance of genetics in the control of the immune response to EBV infection has been established by Purtillo *et al.* (1977) in the X-linked lymphoproliferative syndrome. The ability to identify human leukocyte antigens (HLA) and increasing knowledge of the genetic loci through which they operate may contribute greatly to our future knowledge of "the third ingredient," provided we can compare persons who are known to be infected with controls who are matched in all risk factors and from which group the immune and unexposed can be excluded.

Viruses and Cancer

How can a "third ingredient" be identified in the virus–cancer relationship? The three leading candidates for producing a human cancer—EBV, herpes simplex type 2 (HSV-2), and hepatitis B virus (HBV)*—are ubiquitous agents.

---

*Since 1982, when this article first appeared, papillomavirus types 16 and 18 and HTLV-I have emerged as important candidate agents for human cancer (Evans and Mueller, 1990).

Infection with them is very common in the settings where the cancers are most common. The presence or absence of antibody may thus be difficult to interpret in relation to causation, since both cases and controls have antibody. In EBV-related malignancies the antibody titer has been significantly higher in cases than in healthy controls. This has been shown for over 80% of cases of both African Burkitt's lymphoma (ABL) and nasopharyngeal cancer (NPC) and for 30–40% of Hodgkin's cases. Initially, it was not known whether these results were due to viral multiplication in the tumor itself, to the immunosuppressive therapy given for it, or to an etiological role for the virus. There are several epidemiological approaches to this dilemma. One is to demonstrate that EBV infection and high EBV antibody titers (but not titers of other viral antibodies) preceded the disease, and, thus, might be involved in its pathogenesis. This type of prospective serological study has been done for EBV antibody titers in ABL (de The *et al.*, 1978), Hodgkin's disease (Evans and Comstock, 1981; Mueller *et al.*, 1989) and NPC (Ho *et al.*, 1978; Lamei *et al.*, 1980; Yi *et al.*, 1980). In the ABL study, 42,000 children were bled, among whom 31 cases of tumor developed over a five-year period. Pretumor sera were available for 14 of these. The EBV VCA-IgG antibody titer was equal or higher than in controls in 10 of the 14 ABL cases in serum samples obtained 7 to 54 months *before* the tumor was diagnosed (de The *et al.*, 1978). Other herpes and viral antibody titers were *not* elevated. There was a 30-fold increased risk of later Burkitt tumor development in healthy persons with a 2-fold or greater EBV antibody titer over controls. In another study, two cases of Hodgkin's disease developed among 26,000 normal persons who had been bled in Washington County, Maryland, and whose sera had been stored (Evans and Comstock, 1981). EBV antibodies were uniquely and significantly elevated over controls in sera from these two persons obtained 12 and 21 months prior to diagnosis as compared with four age/sex-matched controls for each. This has been confirmed in a later study of 43 Hodgkin's cases and matched controls (Mueller *et al.*, 1989). In other studies, elevated EBV IgA antibody titers have been shown in three individuals $2\frac{1}{2}$ to 5 years before diagnosis of NPC (Ho *et al.*, 1978), in one of seven Alaskans who subsequently developed NPC (Lamei *et al.*, 1980), and in two Chinese who developed NPC 10 months later (Yi *et al.*, 1980). More recently, massive screening studies for NPC using EBV-IgA antibody as the screening method have been carried out on over 300,000 healthy adults in high-risk areas for the tumor in China (Zeng *et al.*, 1986). The presence of this antibody has not only indicated the possible presence of the tumor, as later confirmed on clinical and biopsy examination, but has also been observed to antedate the appearance of the malignancy by as long as ten years. The presence of elevated antibody titers prior to illness certainly does not establish that the virus necessarily caused the tumor, but it does suggest that it may have played a role directly or indirectly in its pathogenesis.

A second epidemiological approach is to study those persons already possessing high EBV antibody levels to determine if a "third ingredient" can be identified that results in the malignancy. In ABL an added factor is clearly needed to account for the geographic, seasonal, and temporal aspects of the tumor. Most evidence suggests that holoendemic malaria plays this role. EBV has been termed the "initiator" and malaria "the promoter" in this tumor. However, holoendemic malaria is, like EBV, an almost universal infection in early life in this setting. Its occurrence alone would be unlikely to account for ABL in persons so widely infected with both agents, unless strong quantitative differences in the intensity of parasitemia could be shown. Some other ingredient must be inducing the tumor in those who are doubly infected. The search for it is the epidemiological challenge now. In areas where NPC flourishes, EBV infection is also almost universal (de The *et al.*, 1991). Here genetics has been shown to play a role because the highest incidence of the tumor occurs in Chinese living in, or derived from, southern China. In addition, there is almost a fivefold increased risk of NPC among Chinese themselves in the presence of certain HLA configurations (HL-A2, SIN2) as compared with Chinese without these HLA characteristics. In one study, the combination of high-risk Cantonese Chinese and the presence of the HLA characteristics resulted in a 30- to 40-fold higher incidence in this group than in the population of India (de The *et al.*, 1991). Thus, high EBV-IgA antibody levels and genetic background certainly set the stage for NPC, but what third ingredient results in the tumor?

In Hodgkin's disease, prior tonsillectomy, socioeconomic and educational levels, birth order, prior infectious mononucleosis, and elevated EBV antibody titers have been incriminated as important risk factors. However, these risk factors have not been compared in persons with or without high EBV antibody titers to determine if one of them might represent the third ingredient. Recent studies have shown that EBV antibody elevations *precede* the disease and that EBV genome or DNA is present in over 50% of tumor cells in Hodgkin's disease (Mueller *et al.*, 1985; Evans and Mueller, 1990).

Thus, the epidemiological approach to "the third ingredient" in EBV-related malignancies is to compare persons with the malignancy with those persons who have *all* of the pertinent risk factors of the case, including high EBV antibody levels, but who do not have the tumor. Other viral candidates that will require similar investigations are human papillomavirus types 16 and 18 in relation to cervical and vulvar cancer, HBV in relation to hepatocellular cancer, CMV in relation to Kaposi's sarcoma and prostatic cancer, and retroviruses (HTLV-I) in relation to leukemia.

Viruses and Chronic Disease

The role of viruses in the pathogenesis of certain chronic diseases is being increasingly recognized. These involve chronic diseases of the central nervous system (kuru, Creutzfeldt–Jakob disease, subacute sclerosing panencephalitis, progressive multifocal leukoencephalopathy, multiple sclerosis, and allied neurological diseases), of the connective tissues and arteries (systemic lupus erythematosus, sarcoidosis, periarteritis nodosa, rheumatoid arthritis), of the kidney (immune complex nephritis), and of the pancreas (Coxsackie and juvenile diabetes). These exciting advances must be evaluated epidemiologically with methods that recognize susceptibility, infection, and other risk factors in selecting controls. It must be stressed that (1) no one of these putative causes is likely to cause all cases of the disease, (2) other factors ("a third ingredient") are needed in addition to a susceptible host and the putative agent, (3) both the causative agent and the cofactors may be different in different settings without diminishing their important role in causation in a particular setting, and (4) a given agent may operate either directly or indirectly in causation and at different points in the pathogenesis.

Discussion

Advances in molecular virology have yielded very sophisticated techniques to identify the virus, its genome, or its footprints in tissues and to identify particular genome segments that control particular antigenic activities. Second, advances in producing antibody components of high sensitivity and high specificity, particularly the use of monoclonal antibodies, have created a new set of tools to examine the humoral immune response. Third, developments in the study of cell-mediated immunity and its genetic control have permitted a better understanding of the immunoregulation of viral infections. We have learned how this system can both cause and prevent clinical disease. These new virological, immunological, and genetic advances are yielding new insights into disease causation and pathogenesis, and they provide new techniques to the epidemiologist. Causation is increasingly recognized as a multifactorial and complex phenomenon with different sets of risk factors operating in different settings. Many of the causes of disease are so ubiquitous that almost everyone has been exposed to them. This is also true of (direct or indirect) exposures to certain agents, such as tobacco smoke, that are associated with chronic diseases. What then makes disease develop in some who have been exposed, but not in others? It is the search for a clinical illness promotion factor, "a third ingredient," that I urge epidemiologists to pursue. It may be external or internal to the host, it may vary from disease to disease, and it may vary within a single disease in various epidemiological settings. To discover it, one must study a disease intensively within a single ecological setting and compare persons with the disease with exposed and "infected" controls who have all of the same risk markers as the cases. In this effort the epidemiologist should join hands with the virologist, the clinician, the statistician, the immunologist, the biochemist, and the social scientist. If we can identify and modify the clinical illness promotion factor(s), then our efforts at control and prevention can be directed only at those few persons who develop the disease rather than at the total group who are exposed as is our current practice.

References

de The G, Ho JHC, and Muir C: Nasopharyngeal carcinoma, in Evans AS (ed): *Viral Infections of Humans: Epidemiology and Control.* New York, Plenum Press, 1976, pp 539–558.

de The G, Geser A, Day NE, *et al:* Epidemiological evidence for causal relationship between Epstein–Barr virus and Burkitt's lymphoma from Ugandan prospective study. *Nature* **274:**756–761, 1978.

de The G, Ho JHC, Muir C: Nasopharyngeal carcinoma, in Evans AS (ed), *Viral Infections of Humans: Epidemiology and Control,* 3rd ed. New York, Plenum Press, 1991, pp 737–767.

Evans AS: Causation and disease: The Henle–Koch postulates revisited. *Yale J Biol Med* **49:**175–195, 1976.

Evans AS, Comstock GW: Presence of elevated antibody titers to Epstein–Barr virus before Hodgkin's disease. *Lancet* **1:**436, 1981.

Evans AS, Mueller N: Viruses and cancer: Causal associations. *Ann Epidemiol* **1:**71–92, 1990.

Gutensohn N, Cole P: Epidemiology of Hodgkin's disease in the young. *Int J Cancer* **19:**595–604, 1977.

Hallee JT, Evans AS, Niederman JC, *et al:* Infectious mononucleosis at the United States Military Academy. A prospective study of a single class over four years. *Yale J Biol Med* **47:**182–195, 1974.

Henry O: The third ingredient, in *Complete Works of O'Henry.* Garden City, NY, Garden City Publishing Co, 1937, pp 673–682.

Ho HC, Swan HC, Ng MH, *et al:* Serum IgA antibodies to Epstein–Barr capsid antigen preceding symptoms of nasopharyngeal carcinoma. *Lancet* **1:**436, 1978.

Kallman FJ, Reisner D: Twin studies on the significance of genetic factors in tuberculosis. *Am Rev Tuberc* **47:**549–574, 1943.

Kasl SV, Evans AS, Niederman JC, *et al:* Psychosocial risk factors in the development of infectious mononucleosis. *Psychosom Med* **41:**445–466, 1979.

Lamei AP, Henle W, Bender TR, *et al:* Epstein–Barr virus-specific antibody titers in seven Alaskan natives before and after diagnosis of nasopharyngeal carcinoma. *Int J Cancer* **26:**133–138, 1980.

Mueller N, Evans AS, Harris N., *et al:* Hodgkin's disease and Epstein–Barr virus. Evidence of altered antibody pattern prior to diagnosis. *N Engl J Med* **320:**689–695, 1989.

Pan LW: Host variation in the manifestations of disease, with particular reference to homologous serum jaundice in the army of the United States. *Med Ann DC* **14:**443–449, 1945.

Purtillo DT, De Florio D Jr, Hutt LM, *et al:* Variable phenotypic expression of an X-linked recessive lymphoproliferative syndrome. *N Engl J Med* **297:**1077–1081, 1977.

Reedy JJ: Recessive inheritance of susceptibility to poliomyelitis in fifty pedigrees. *J Hered* **48:**37–44, 1957.

Wilson MG, Sweitzer MD: Pattern of hereditary susceptibility in rheumatic fever. *Circulation* **10:**699–704, 1954.

Yi X, Yuxi L, Chunren L, *et al:* Application of an immuno-enzymatic and immunoradiographic method for a mass survey of nasopharyngeal carcinoma. *Intervirology* **13:**162–168, 1980.

12

Subclinical Epidemiology

The occurrence of infection without disease is a well-recognized phenomenon in infectious diseases to which the terms "inapparent" or "subclinical" are usually applied. The known determinants of whether a given infection results in clinical or in subclinical illness have been discussed in the previous chapter. Age at the time of infection is certainly an important host determinant but the mechanism by which this occurs is poorly understood. Some of these factors lie in our immuno-logical system and our genetic makeup but others are unknown and remain a major challenge to investigators. If we could discover these secrets that result in clinical illness in some and in subclinical illness in others, and find a way to modify the host's response so that only the latter results, then we could achieve natural immunity without disease. The characteristics of the agent also play an important role in this phenomenon, to which the terms "pathogenicity" and "virulence" are applied.

The recognition of the presence of an inapparent or subclinical illness in infectious disease depends on criteria such as those outlined in Table 12.1. The demonstration of the infectious agent and/or an immune response to it are critical elements of proof.

While there is wide appreciation of the existence of subclinical illness in infectious diseases, little attention has been devoted to their existence and recog-nition in chronic diseases. As a basis for prevention and control, it is important that the epidemiologist understand the full range of host responses to a set of risk factors because strategies for intervention may differ at different points in the pathogenesis of the disease. This is dependent on a full knowledge of the natural history of a disease.

In this chapter I will present a concept of the steps in this natural history and indicate its application to infectious, chronic, and malignant disease. It is based in large part on an earlier paper of mine on this subject (Evans, 1987); some parts are also repetitious of Chapter 11 but are needed to provide a full explanation of the concept.

My simplified concept involves three phases in the natural history of the

Table 12.1
Criteria for a Subclinical Infection[a]

1. A well-defined clinical syndrome
2. Known and identifiable causes of the syndrome demonstrable by laboratory tests (appearance of antibody, presence of IgM antibody, antigen isolation or identification)
3. The ability to differentiate between the laboratory markers of acute and of past infection
4. The occurrence of subclinical cases concurrently with clinical cases, especially during an epidemic or in close contacts of the subclinical cases

[a]From Evans (1991).

disease process, as shown in Table 12.2. They are: (a) exposure to the risk factors, which are pathogenic in some individuals and invoke no host response in others; (b) factors resulting in the initiation of the pathologic process and/or the markers thereof, both in infectious and in chronic diseases; and (c) factors that lead in some individuals to clinical disease and in others to a subclinical or inapparent illness. I have termed these influences the "clinical illness promotion factors" (Evans, 1985). The late Dr. Bernard Greenberg looked at the same issue from the standpoint of the factors that *prevent* clinical illness (Greenberg, 1983).

Table 12.2
Natural History of Clinical and Subclinical Illness

Exposure	Pathologic process	Clinical/subclinical

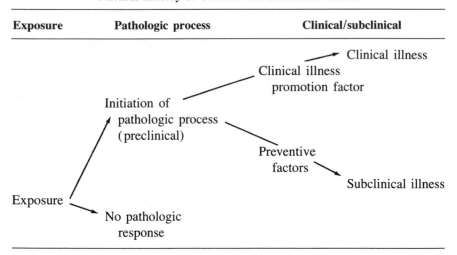

We are both interested in the determinants that result in clinical illness in some persons and in subclinical or inapparent illness in others. The question might be extended further back in the natural history of disease to ask why some adequately exposed persons develop the pathologic process and others escape entirely.

The purposes of preclinical and subclinical epidemiology can be listed as follows:

1. To identify the factors in exposure that are potentially pathogenic for humans and the factors that lead to the pathologic process in some individuals and have no effect in others.
2. To identify the factors in those with the pathologic process that lead to clinical illness in some and to subclinical or inapparent illness in others.
3. To direct preventive and control programs at the susceptible persons and at the factors that lead from exposure to the pathologic process and then to clinical illness.

Prospective, cohort studies that utilize serial laboratory and clinical evaluation of those at risk provide the best means to identify the earliest evidence of the pathologic process among exposed individuals. Table 12.3 presents a statistical expression of the rates in this concept. This model will now be discussed in relation to infectious diseases, coronary heart disease, and certain cancers, giving specific examples wherever possible.

In infectious diseases, the risk factors involved in each of the three steps in pathogenesis are shown in Table 12.4. The determinants of exposure are quite well defined for most infectious diseases as are some of the key factors that lead to the initiation of the pathologic process, which we call "infection." These involve the dosage, duration of exposure, and pathogenicity of the agent and certain key host factors such as the immune status and the immunologic nature of the response. The genetic characteristics of both the agent and the host are often critical elements in the outcome. For example, minor alterations in the bio-

Table 12.3
Statistical Expression of Pathogenetic Process

$$\text{Rate of pathogenetic process} = \frac{\text{Number with pathogenic markers (in infectious disease = infection)}}{\text{Number exposed (and susceptible)}}$$

$$\text{Rate of clinical illness} = \frac{\text{Number with clinical illness}}{\text{Number with pathologic process}}$$

Table 12.4
Risk Factors in Infectious Diseases

Exposure	Pathologic process	Clinical illness
Presence of agent	Dosage and duration	Virulence of agent
Socioeconomic level	Immune status of host	Age when infected
Behavioral factors	Behavioral factors	Behavioral factors
Means of transmission	Presence of receptors	Immune response
Effective contact	Genetic susceptibility	Genetic susceptibility

chemical makeup of several viruses such as the reovirus (Sharpe and Fields, 1985) can determine whether infection will occur, the severity of the illness produced, and even the pattern of the host response; a change in a single nucleotide of rabies virus renders it avirulent (Notkins, 1985). But even when exposed to the same agent, genetic characteristics of the host are also determinants of the host's response and of the immunologic mechanisms involved in both protection and pathogenicity. Genetic susceptibility also probably plays a key role at several stages in the pathogenesis of chronic and malignant diseases. The technology needed to identify the genetically susceptible person is difficult, but, in addition to the classical studies of twins, the use of DNA recombinant technology and of genetic linkage using DNA probes now permit identification of the responsible gene and in a few diseases even to clone it [e.g., in the case of Huntington's chorea (Martin and Gusella, 1986), Tay–Sachs disease (Gusella *et al.*, 1984), Duchenne muscular dystrophy, and retinoblastoma (Kolata, 1986)]. As regards infectious diseases, we have good markers for *infection* such as the appearance of antibody or of a positive skin test and the isolation and/or identification of the agent. Advances in molecular biology for antigen detection and in monoclonal antibody technology for diagnosis have resulted in highly sensitive and specific tools. We are less certain of the clinical illness promotion factors (Evans, 1982) that result in manifest illness among some of those infected and the protective factors (Greenberg, 1983) that lead to subclinical illness in others. In most viral and bacterial infections, this latter group constitutes the great majority of infected persons (exceptions include rabies and measles). We are currently seeking such answers in those infected with the human immunodeficiency virus (HIV) [human T-cell lymphotropic virus type III/lymphadenopathy-associated virus (HTLV-III/LAV)], the causative agent of AIDS, using prospective seroepidemiologic studies.

We have pursued this same methodology in studying the development of Epstein–Barr virus (EBV) infection and its clinical manifestation, infectious mononucleosis, in a cohort of about 1400 cadets over 4 years at the West Point Military Academy (Hallee *et al.*, 1974). Of the total groups, 63% were immune on entry into the academy, as shown by the presence of EBV antibody. Of the 432 susceptible cadets lacking this antibody, 194 (44.9%) became infected over the 4-year period and 238 were still susceptible at the time of graduation. While the degree, intensity, and multiplicity of exposure, as manifested by intimate oral contact, may have varied from person to person and the likelihood of kissing an EBV excretor was about one in five, these do not seem adequate explanations why this latter group of cadets escaped infection. Among the 194 cadets who became infected, as demonstrated by seroconversion on serial sampling, 48 (24.7%) developed clinical infectious mononucleosis and the other 75.3% had subclinical illness.

We were interested in the determinants of these outcomes. An intensive psychosocial evaluation carried out at the time of entry for another reason provided clues to certain clinical illness promotion factors when correlated with the results of our data on susceptibility, infection, and disease associated with EBV, as shown in Table 12.5. The key factors were (1) having a father who was an

Table 12.5

Relation of Degree of Commitment to a Military Career and Relative Academic Performance during the 3rd and 4th Year as a Risk Factor for Clinical Infectious Mononucleosis (IM) among West Point Military Academy Cadets Infected with Epstein–Barr Virus (EBV) during the Study Period[a]

Risk factor	No. of cadets	% developing clinical IM among those infected with EBV in 2nd and 3rd year
Commitment to a military career		
Low	28	10.7
Moderate	145	22.8
High	21	57.1
Total	194	24.7
Academic performance: 2nd semester grades		
Worse than 1st semester	16	50.0
About same as 1st semester	21	23.8
Better than 1st semester	18	5.6

[a]Table derived from data in Kasl *et al.* (1979). The differences shown were statistically significant but no significant difference was seen in academic performance and IM in 2nd year grades and those predicted from background data.

overachiever, (2) having a high level of motivation, and (3) doing relatively poorly academically. For example, cadets who received poorer marks in the second semester of their third and fourth year at the academy than in the first semester had a 50% rate of clinical infectious mononucleosis following infection, compared with a rate of 5% among those who did better in the second semester. High motivation and poor academic performance taken together were good predictors of clinical illness among the infected. These factors also predicted the development of heterophile antibody in cadets with subclinical illness and the length of hospitalization among those with infectious mononucleosis. These objective observations diminished the possibility that the findings were due to the cadet's perception of illness or willingness to seek medical care. Thus, the serious, highly motivated student who had an overachieving father and who was not doing well academically was less likely to be infected either before or after entry into the academy, but once infected had a much higher chance of developing clinical illness than his more easygoing and more exposed counterpart. If one had focused on a case–control study of clinical illness without knowledge of susceptibility on entry and of the infection rate, the behavioral pattern would have been obscured. These studies are compatible with the earlier observations of Greenfield et al. (1959) that ego-strength influenced the duration of clinical infectious mononucleosis, and those of Clough et al. (1966) on the incidence of clinical influenza in psychologically "vulnerable" and "non-vulnerable" persons. They are examples of the use of laboratory and psychologic markers to define factors that influence clinical illness. I hope that such markers can be applied to other infectious diseases as well as to chronic diseases.

The effect of genetic background on the development of clinical tuberculosis among susceptible persons (i.e., persons with negative skin tests) who were exposed to an index case in a family setting was well shown by Kallman and Reisner (1943) (Table 12.6). The risk of developing clinical tuberculosis among those infected after exposure varied directly with the degree of genetic relatedness.

Similarly, a study by Van Eden et al. (1983) to determine the level at which genetic factors might operate in the development of infection and/or clinical disease in poliomyelitis has indicated that the effect is among those infected who go on to develop paralytic disease and not on the rate of infection among those exposed. Purtillo et al. (1977) have shown that genetic regulation of the immune response also plays a role in the various clinical expressions of EBV infection in the X-linked lymphoproliferative syndrome. These early leads offer the hope that we may be able to identify persons who are susceptible to infection and persons who are susceptible to disease and thus direct our preventive approaches to a smaller and more specific population and at a more efficient level in the natural history of the disease process.

In chronic diseases, the risk factors of exposure are often more difficult to

Table 12.6
Effect of Genetic Relatedness on Host Response
to *M. tuberculosis* in Families
with an Index Case[a]

Relation of family member to index case	% of exposed and susceptibles showing clinical manifestations of tuberculosis
Marriage partner	7.1
Half-sibling	11.9
Dizygotic twin	25.5
Monozygotic twin	83.3

[a]Table derived from data in Kallman and Reisner (1943).

ascertain and the markers of the early pathologic process have not been well defined for many diseases, so that no denominator of "infected" may be available. This explains the popularity of the case–control study, which takes, as a starting point, cases of the disease in order to identify risk factors for the disease. The intermediate steps of how many of those exposed develop the pathologic process and how many develop the clinical illness are unknown. Some of the factors involved in the development of coronary heart disease are depicted in Table 12.7. Exposure includes dietary, behavioral (Type A personality), and genetic factors, accompanied by a stressful, sedentary life-style and cigarette smoking. Persons with high blood pressure, impaired glucose tolerance, high cholesterol, an increase in low-density lipoprotein (LDL) cholesterol, and/or a decrease in high-density lipoprotein (HDL) cholesterol, and with genetic defects that result in a deficiency of liver receptors that process LDL cholesterol, can be regarded as being "infected," i.e., the pathologic process is under way. It is not clear what factors among this group lead to clinical coronary disease in some persons and subclinical illness in others. However, the duration and intensity of the pathogenetic factors must be important. LDL cholesterol seems to be a clinical illness promoter and HDL cholesterol a preventive factor; genetics and family history and stress are probably involved. Of these persons falling into the upper 20% of the major risk factors (high blood pressure, smoking, high total cholesterol, and high LDL cholesterol), some 50% will develop a coronary disease event in the next 8 years (Kannel *et al.*, 1984; W. B. Kannel, personal communication, 1986). So one challenge is to find out why persons in that 50% are at risk to clinical illness and the other 50% are not. Indeed, it appears that only about 50–70% of the cases of coronary heart disease are explicable by the

Table 12.7
Risk Factors in Coronary Heart Disease[a]

Exposure	Pathologic process	Clinical illness
Dietary		
High cholesterol	High total cholesterol	Angina pectoris
Unsaturated fats	High LDL cholesterol	Myocardial infarction
Overeating	Genetic susceptibility	Sudden death
Cigarette smoking	Cigarette smoking	Angina pectoris and infarction
Lack of exercise	Glucose intolerance	Diabetes
Stress	Behavioral (Type A personality)	Behavioral (Type A personality)
Family environment	Increased risk factors	Increased illness
Oral contraceptives		
		Subclinical illness
		Electrocardiographic changes on exercise
		Left ventricular hypertrophy

[a]About half of the persons with high blood pressure and high LDL and total cholesterol, who smoke cigarettes, will develop a coronary disease event in the next eight years (Kannel *et al.*, 1984, W. B. Kannel, personal communication, 1986).

known risk factors, much like the status of our etiologic knowledge of some of the common clinical syndromes in infectious diseases. A second challenge is to identify the other risk factors involved in the pathogenesis of coronary heart disease. Dr. William B. Kannel, Director of the Framingham prospective heart study, has a concept of the pathogenesis of coronary heart disease based on four categories of risk elements, as shown in Table 12.8. These categories are similar to those discussed here but are arranged in a somewhat different order and fashion. We share the belief that the identification and protection of those at highest risk is our major challenge. Some factors appear to operate at several levels in pathogenesis, such as smoking and obesity. It is encouraging that some of these factors are not only reversible but that there has been a big drop in coronary artery deaths and in stroke in the United States over the past few years (Kannel *et al.*, 1984). Dietary changes, cessation of smoking, and more vigorous exercise have all contributed to this decline (Kannel *et al.*, 1984). Some obvious and some theoretical approaches to prevention are listed in Table 12.9.

Cancer is the third major disease category I wish to discuss. Here the term

Table 12.8
Classes of Cardiovascular Risk Factors[a]

1. Living habits: Overeating; lack of exercise; cigarette smoking. Type A behavior (?)
2. Atherogenic personal attributes: High blood pressure; hyperglycemia; dyslipidemia; elevated fibrinogen.
3. Indicators of compromised circulation: Electrocardiographic abnormalities at rest; on exercise; on ambulatory monitoring; vascular bruits; echocardiographic abnormalities; myocardial perfusion deficits, etc.
4. Host susceptibility: Inborn errors of metabolism; family history of premature cardiovascular disease.

[a]Table derived from Kannel and Lerner (1984), Kannel et al. (1984), and W. B. Kannel (personal communication, 1986).

"initiator(s)" is used to indicate the risk factor or factors implicated in the genesis of the pathologic or oncogenic process and the term "promoter" for the factor or factors that lead to the development of the clinical tumor. Certainly, lung cancer is an excellent example of smoking as the initiator of the pathologic process. But what is the promoter that leads to cancer in some 10% of persons who smoke two packs of cigarettes a day over 20 years and/or what is the protective factor that lets the other 90% escape? There is recent evidence that genetic susceptibility may have an important role in this and that certain persons

Table 12.9
Heart Disease: Approaches to Prevention

Exposure	Pathogenesis	Clinical illness
Better diet	Lower cholesterol with drugs	Coronary bypass
	Extract HDL from blood	Blow out clot
	Add LDL receptors (?)	Dissolve clot
Stop smoking	Stop smoking	Stop smoking
Reduce stress	Reduce stress	Reduce stress
Exercise	Exercise	Carefully controlled exercise
Identify genetic susceptibles to: Obesity Liver lipid receptors		

are able to detoxify the oncogenic components in cigarette smoke and others are not (K. K. Kidd, personal communication, 1986). Knowledge of the stage of action of the risk factors is critical for a proper understanding of the pathogenesis and prevention of this and other malignancies.

African Burkitt's lymphoma is an example of the use of laboratory techniques in studying the pathogenesis of a malignancy. Prospective seroepidemiologic studies, as carried out by de The *et al.* (1978), permit a portrayal of the natural history of the lymphoma, as depicted in Table 12.10. This table also shows the course of nasopharyngeal carcinoma based on screening tests carried out for IgA antibody to EBV in some 50,000 Chinese persons in an endemic area by Yi *et al.* (1980) (see discussion below). In African Burkitt's lymphoma, exposure to EBV in infancy, the initiation of B-cell proliferation by the virus, and the promoting effect of repeated malarial infection appear to be key events resulting in a chromosomal shift from 8 to 14 (or, less commonly, to chromosome 2 or 22) and the emergence of the malignant cell that makes Burkitt's lymphoma a monoclonal malignancy. Events at the molecular level involving the activation of the c-*myc* oncogene, the transfer of an immunoglobulin regulator from one chromosome to another, and the possible role of two other oncogenes (H-*ras* and B-*lym*) have been implicated in the pathogenesis of the tumor (Leder, 1985a,b). Genetic susceptibility may be another determinant of whether the clinical tumor will develop or not, as indicated by the finding of Jones *et al.* (1985) that persons with HLA-DR7 had a relative risk of 3.7 for the tumor as compared with matched controls without this marker. Since EBV infection early in life and repeated malarial infections appear to involve the entire population, almost all can be regarded as infected and subject to the initiation of the pathologic process, as manifested by the proliferation of B cells, and, in some persons, an increase in antibodies to the viral capsid antigen of EBV. Since the markers of recent infection (IgM antibody and early antigen antibody increases) are not also elevated at this time, an acute and/or persistent infection does not seem to be part of the process. However, the elevated IgG titer creates a new denominator of risk such that persons with titers two or more dilutions higher than control children have a 30-fold increase in risk to the clinical tumor. Because all sera were not tested for antibody levels, we don't know the absolute risk of tumor in those with high titers. It may be on the order of 30–40%, thus making the occurrence of tumor a rare event, given a large denominator. It also seems possible that not every person who develops the chromosomal shift will go on to develop Burkitt's lymphoma, perhaps because of cell death. On the other hand, however, all cases of the tumor studied have shown one of the three characteristic chromosomal shifts. In the end, about one in 3000 children followed developed Burkitt's lymphoma. If we are able to define these risk factors for tumor development more accurately, then we have tools to seek early diagnosis and perhaps initiate protective measures. But while EBV and malaria may be the initiators in Africa,

Table 12.10

Postulated Pathogenesis of the Role of Epstein–Barr Virus (EBV) in African Burkitt's Lymphoma (ABL) and Nasopharyngeal Cancer (NPC) in China[a]

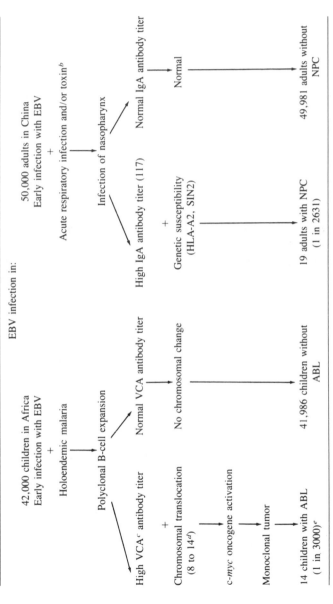

[a]Table derived from data in de The *et al.* (1978) and Yi *et al.* (1980).
[b]Toxin might be tung oil or other phorbol ester and reactivated virus rather than the initial nasopharyngeal infection.
[c]VCA, viral capsid antigen.
[d]Less commonly, translocation is to chromosome 2 or 22.
[e]Of the 14 cases of ABL, 10 had twofold or higher titers to EBV-VCA antibody than controls.

Burkitt's lymphoma in the United States is related to high EBV antibody in only about one-third of the cases: some 20% lack the antibody altogether, and malaria is nonexistent. So other risk factors must be operative (Evans, 1985). This means that the etiologic factors may vary from place to place and involve different strategies for control.

In China, EBV infection also occurs early in life (Wang and Evans, 1986), but nasopharyngeal cancer appears in the adult. EBV IgA antibody as an indicator of the start of the pathologic process is depicted using data from the study by Yi *et al.* (1980), on the right side of Table 12.10. Of about 50,000 adults tested in an endemic area for the tumor, 117 persons were found to have EBV IgA antibody in their serum and subsequent examination of this group revealed 19 persons to have nasopharyngeal cancer. What factors determined the development of IgA antibody? Was it some activator such as tung oil or some other phorbol ester known to activate EBV in B lymphocytes? Or was it nitrosamines in smoked fish that made the tumor cell permissive to EBV infection? And of the group with IgA antibody, why did only 19 out of 117 persons show the tumor? Perhaps some of the others will manifest it later since two have already done so in the 2 years following the initial examination.

Finally, the fine prospective study of Beasley *et al.* (1981) is another example of the use of laboratory methods in understanding the development of a malignancy, in this instance the relation to hepatitis B virus infection and the later emergence of hepatocellular cancer. The results of their study are summarized in Table 12.11. A cohort of some 23,000 young men in Taiwan was followed, of which 3454 (15%) had hepatitis B antigenemia and the rest did not. Among the antigenemic group, 40 developed primary hepatocellular carcinoma, in contrast

Table 12.11
Results of Follow-up of 22,707 Men for an Average Period of 3.3 Years for Deaths Due to Primary Hepatocellular Carcinoma (PHC), Cirrhosis, or Other Causes in Taiwan, According to Hepatitis B Surface Antigen (HBsAg) Status on Entry into Study[a]

| HBsAg status on entry | No. in Category | Cause of death | | | PHC incidence[b] |
		PHC	Cirrhosis	Other	
HBsAg-positive	3,454	40	17	48	1158 } RR[c] = 223
HBsAg-negative	19,253	1	2	199	5
Total	22,707	41	19	247	181

[a]Table adapted from data in Beasley *et al.* (1981)
[b]Incidence of death from PHC per 100,000 during time of study.
[c]RR, relative risk.

to only 2 in the antigen-negative group, a relative risk of 223. But why did only 1 in 86 with antigenemia develop hepatocellular carcinoma and the rest escape? These observations have now led to trials to prevent early infection by hepatitis B virus using active and/or passive immunization of newborn infants in the hope of avoiding the later development of the tumor. If this turns out to be the case, it will be the first human cancer preventable by immunization.

In summary, the suggestion is made that epidemiological studies of infectious, chronic, and malignant diseases use laboratory methods to identify the initiation of the pathologic process following exposure and then to search for the factors in such persons that lead to clinical illness in some persons and to mild or subclinical illness in others. If we can define these subsets of risk in the natural history of disease, then we can focus our preventive and control programs on those who are truly exposed and susceptible.

References

Beasley P, Hwang L-Y, Lin C-C, et al: Hepatocellular carcinoma and hepatitis B virus. A prospective study of 22,107 men in Taiwan. *Lancet* **2**:1129–1133, 1981.

Clough L, Canter A, Imboden JB: Asian influenza. Infection, disease, and psychological factors. *Arch Intern Med* **117**:159–163, 1966.

de The G, Geser A, Day NE, et al: Epidemiological evidence of causal relationship between Epstein–Barr virus and Burkitt's lymphoma from Ugandan prospective study. *Nature* **274**:756–761, 1978.

Evans AS: The clinical illness promotion factor. A third ingredient. *Yale J Biol Med* **55**:193–199, 1982.

Evans AS: Epidemiology of Burkitt's lymphoma; other risk factors, in Lenoir G, O'Conor G, Olweny CLM (eds): *Burkitt's Lymphoma: A Human Cancer Model.* IARC Scientific Publication No. 60. Lyons, IARC, 1985, pp 197–204.

Evans AS: Subclinical epidemiology. *Am J Epidemiol* **125**:545–555, 1987.

Evans AS: Chronic fatigue syndrome: Thoughts on pathogenesis. *Rev Infect Dis* **13**(suppl 1): S56–S59, 1991.

Greenberg B: The future of epidemiology. *J Chronic Dis* **361**:353–359, 1983.

Greenfield NS, Roessler R, Crosley AP Jr: Ego strength and length of recovery from infectious mononucleosis. *J Nerv Ment Dis* **128**:125–128, 1959.

Gusella JF, Tangi RE, Anderson MA, et al: DNA markers for nervous system diseases. *Science* **225**:1320–1326, 1984.

Hallee TJ, Evans AS, Niederman JC: Infectious mononucleosis at the United States Military Academy. A prospective study of a single class over four years. *Yale J Biol Med* **3**:182–195, 1974.

Jones EH, Biggar RJ, Nkrumah, et al: HLA-DR7 association with African Burkitt's lymphoma. *Hum Immunol* **13**:211–217, 1985.

Kallman FJ, Reisner D: Twin studies on the genetic factors in tuberculosis. *Am Rev Tuberc* **47**:549–574, 1943.

Kannel WB, Lerner DJ: Present status of risk factors for atherosclerosis. *Med Times* **112**:33–45, 1984.

Kannel WB, Doyle JT, Ostfeld AM, *et al:* Optimal resources for primary prevention of atherosclerotic diseases: Atherosclerotic Study Group. *Circulation* **70:**157A–205A, 1984.

Kasl SV, Evans AS, Niederman JC: Psychosocial risk factors in the development of infectious mononucleosis. *Psychosom Med* **41:**445–465, 1979.

Kolata G: Two disease-causing genes found. *Science* **234:**669–670, 1986.

Leder P: Translocation among antibody genes in human cancer, in Lenoir G, O'Conor G, Olweny CLM (eds): *Burkitt's Lymphoma: A Human Cancer Model.* IARC Publication No. 60. Lyons, IARC, 1985a, pp 341–357.

Leder P: The state and prospects for molecular genetics, in Lenoir G, O'Conor G, Olweny CLM (eds): *Burkitt's Lymphoma: A Human Cancer Model.* IARC Publication No. 60. Lyons, IARC, 1985b, pp 475–476.

Martin JB, Gusella JF: Huntington's disease: Pathogenesis and management. *N Engl J Med* **315:**1267–1276, 1986.

Notkins AL: (Editorial) Molecular biology and viral pathogenesis. Clinical spinoff. *N Engl J Med* **312:**507–509, 1985.

Purtillo DT, de Florio D Jr, Hutt LM, *et al:* Variable phenotypic expression of an X-linked recessive lymphoproliferative syndrome. *N Engl J Med* **297:**1077–1081, 1977.

Sharpe AH, Fields BN: Pathogenesis of viral infections: Basic concepts derived from the reovirus model. *N Engl J Med* **312:**486–496, 1985.

Van Eden W, Persijn GG, Bijkerk H, *et al:* Differential resistance to paralytic poliomyelitis controlled by histocompatibility leukocyte antigens. *J Infect Dis* **147:**422–426, 1983.

Wang P-SD, Evans AS: Prevalence of antibodies to Epstein–Barr virus in sera from a group of children in the Republic of China. *J Infect Dis* **153:**150–152, 1986.

Yi Z, Yuxi L, Chunren L, *et al:* Application of a method for mass survey of nasopharyngeal carcinoma. *Intervirology* **13:**162–168, 1980.

Epilogue

This monograph has reviewed our changing concepts of the causation of disease. Perhaps it is time that we also look at the causation of health (Table 1). Let us direct our attention not only to those factors that produce disease but also to those that produce health. Let us change our "don'ts" for "dos" in medical practice and public health. Some of the possible "dos" are listed in Table 2. They include both health and social suggestions. The evidence that these factors play a role in keeping us healthy needs scientific validation. The nature of the studies will be the opposite of those currently run. We will be seeking "clues to health" rather than illness. Case–control studies will focus on the healthy person as the "case" and the ill person as the control. Prospective or cohort studies will be concerned with the factors that keep the healthy persons in good health rather than those that make us ill. We must recognize that there will be multiple causes of "health" just as there are multiple causes of a disease. These risk factors for health will not

Table 1
Postulates for the Causation of Health

1. The preventive factor must be consistently present in persons of good health or free of a particular disease.
2. The factor must be isolable in a pure form (i.e., can be identified as causal).
3. The extent to which the factor is effectively applied must parallel an increase in good health and/or freedom from that disease.
4. Experimental application of the factor to one segment of a population should significantly increase their good health as compared with matched controls.
5. Withdrawal of the preventive factor should be associated with an increase of disease associated with that factor.
6. The effect of the factor shall be measured in terms of lower morbidity and mortality, longer life, and lower medical costs.

Table 2
Possible "Dos" in Health

Exercise daily and moderately.
Take modest amounts of alcohol daily.
Take an aspirin a day.
Take life easy.
Be a Type B personality.
Eat a low-fat diet.
Eat three normal meals daily.
Get six to seven hours sleep nightly.
Get faith and equanimity.

---

only be more numerous than those of disease but will also be more diverse. The World Health Organization has defined health as follows:

> Health is a state of complete physical, mental, and social well-being and not merely the absence of disease or infirmity.

Thus, the risk factors will include not only physical and mental factors but also social factors. The challenge to the epidemiologist is to define which of these are most important, the extent to which each contributes to health (relative risk), and the cost–benefit ratio in attaining that goal. It should also be emphasized that there is a "biological spectrum of health" just as there is one of disease. This might range in the iceberg concept from "just getting by without illness" to the peak, the "complete" attainment included in the WHO definition. The individual level of "health" will vary from one society to another, from one individual to another, and for each individual according to age, sex, education, and socioeconomic status.

Our daily television, radio, newspaper, and magazine advertisements besiege us with various nostrums to keep us healthy or make us healthier ranging from vitamin pills, to "Geritol," to mouthwashes, to exercise machines. It is time we, as scientists and as epidemiologists, start conducting "clinical trials" to establish the efficacy of these factors. We must recognize that establishing the factors promoting health and the proof of causation of health will be more difficult and more challenging than the causation of disease. But let us begin.

Index